Dyspepsia

For a catalogue of publications available from ACP–ASIM, contact:

Customer Service Center
American College of Physicians–American Society of Internal Medicine
190 N. Independence Mall West
Philadelphia, PA 19106-1572
215-351-2600
800-523-1546, ext. 2600

Visit our Web site at www.acponline.org

Dyspepsia

■ ■ ■

David A. Johnson, MD, FACP, FACG
Professor of Medicine
Eastern Virginia Medical School
Norfolk, Virginia

Philip O. Katz, MD, FACP, FACG
Associate Professor of Medicine
MCP–Hahnemann School of Medicine
Chief of Gastroenterology and Vice Chairman, Medicine
Graduate Hospital
Philadelphia, Pennsylvania

Donald O. Castell, MD, FACP, FACG
Kimble Professor of Medicine and Chairman
Department of Medicine
MCP–Hahnemann School of Medicine
Graduate Hospital
Philadelphia, Pennsylvania

A|C|P

American College of Physicians
Philadelphia, Pennsylvania

Clinical Consultant: David R. Goldmann, MD
Manager, Book Publishing: David Myers
Administrator, Book Publishing: Diane McCabe
Production Supervisor: Allan S. Kleinberg
Production Editor: Scott Thomas Hurd
Developmental Editor: Victoria Hoenigke
Acquisitions Editor: Mary K. Ruff
Editorial Assistant: Alicia Dillihay
Interior Design: Kate Nichols
Cover Design: Elizabeth Swartz
Indexer: Nelle Garrecht

Printed in the United States of America
Composition by Fulcrum Data Services, Inc.
Printing/binding by Versa Press

American College of Physicians (ACP) became an imprint of the American College of Physicians–American Society of Internal Medicine in July 1998.

Library of Congress Cataloging-in-Publication Data

Dyspepsia / [edited by] David A. Johnson, Philip O. Katz, Donald O. Castell.
   p.; cm. -- (ACP Key diseases series)
   Includes bibliographical references and index.
   ISBN 0-943126-97-5
   1. Indigestion. I. Johnson, David A., 1954– II. Katz, Philip O., 1953– III. Castell,
Donald O. IV. Series.
   [DNLM: 1. Dyspepsia--diagnosis. 2. Dyspepsia--therapy. 3. Diagnosis, Differential.
   4. Evidence-Based Medicine. WI145 D9978 2000]
   RC827.R972 2000
   616.3'32--dc21   00-044765

01 02 03 04 05 / 9 8 7 6 5 4 3 2 1

Contributors

Brooks D. Cash, MD
Assistant Professor of Medicine
Uniformed Services University of the
    Health Sciences
F. Edward Herbert School of Medicine
Bethesda, Maryland

Hartley Cohen, MD, FACP
Professor of Medicine
Department of Medicine
Division of Gastroenterology
USC School of Medicine
Los Angeles, California

Kenneth R. DeVault, MD, FACG
Associate Professor of Medicine
Mayo Clinic Jacksonville
Jacksonville, Florida

A. Mark Fendrick, MD
Associate Professor, Internal Medicine,
    Health Management and Policy
School of Public Health
University of Michigan School of
    Medicine
Ann Arbor, Michigan

M. Brian Fennerty, MD
Associate Professor of Medicine
Section Chief, Gastroenterology
OHSU Division of
    Gastroenterology/Hepatology
Portland, Oregon

Loren Laine, MD
Professor of Medicine
Department of Medicine
Division of Gastroenterology
USC School of Medicine
Los Angeles, California

**Darryl Mackender, MB, BS(Syd),
    FRACP, MPH**
Gosford Hospital
Gosford, New South Wales, Australia

Joshua J. Ofman, MD, MSHS
Assistant Professor of Medicine,
    Vice President of Research
Cedars-Sinai Departments of Medicine
    and Health Services Research
Division of Gastroenterology
Zynx Health, Inc.
Beverly Hills, California

Walter L. Peterson, MD, FACP
Professor of Internal Medicine
University of Texas Southwestern
    Medical School at Dallas
Dallas, Texas

Eammon M.M. Quigley, MD, FRCP
Professor of Medicine
National University of Ireland, Cork
Department of Medicine
Cork University Hospital
Cork, Ireland

**Philip Schoenfeld, MD, MSEd,
    MSc(Epi)**
National Naval Medical Center
Division of Gastroenterology
Uniformed Services University of the
    Health Sciences
Bethesda, Maryland

Nicholas J. Talley, MD, PhD, FACP
Professor of Medicine
University of Western Sydney
Nepean Hospital
Nepean, New South Wales, Australia

Contents

Introduction

The term *dyspepsia* represents a variety of symptoms pertaining to the upper gastrointestinal tract, inlcuding upper abdominal pain, discomfort, heartburn, nausea, bloating, and regurgitation. Typically, physicians attempt to classify dyspepsia patients by symptom pattern or suspected underlying disease, which has led to qualified diagnoses, such as "reflux-like," "ulcer-like," "dysmotility-like," and "nonulcer, nonspecific" dyspepsia. The symptom pattern and response to empirical therapy are helpful in establishing the specific classification.

When examining dyspepsia patients, the physician must distinguish between organic and functional causes of dyspepsia. This can be established typically by directed investigation via endoscopy, radiography, or laboratory tests. However, an empirical approach to therapy has had increasing appeal, and a response to empirical therapy is now viewed by many experts as a diagnostic test in and of itself. The prevalence of dyspepsia is estimated to be as high as 26% in the United States (1). Although only 20% to 25% of patients with dyspepsia reportedly seek medical care, dyspeptic complaints are responsible for 2% to 5% of visits to primary care physicians (2), resulting in substantial health care costs, both on a direct and indirect basis. Direct costs include specific physician visits, diagnostic testing, and pharmacologic intervention. Indirect costs include absenteeism, altered effectiveness in the workplace, and quality-of-life implications.

The diagnosis of dyspepsia in itself has significant cost implications. Endoscopic and radiologic evaluations can be quite costly, and newer technologies will likely be even more expensive. The ultimate goal of the physician, however, is to balance the appropriate diagnostic strategy with the optimal use of health care resources. Similarly, the appropriate use of medical therapy should always focus on the medication that achieves the best symptomatic response. It is becoming increasingly well recognized that no or poor treatment of upper gastrointestinal visceral diseases has a significant effect on qualify of life. Therefore, attempting to use the *least costly* medication may seem like an idealistic goal, but the therapeutic tradeoff may be using one that is *less effective*. Clearly, the most expensive therapy is the one that does not work and leads to continued costs due to diagnostic testing or escalating medication requirements (3,4).

Several other factors introduce major questions about the diagnostic management strategies for dyspepsia. The exploration of information on *Helicobacter pylori* clearly has complicated management strategies (outside the standard patients with peptic ulcer disease). Furthermore, growing data on empirical therapies with proton-pump inhibitors, appropriate prokinetic agents, "safer" nonsteroidal anti-inflammatory drugs (e.g., Cox-2 inhibitors), and over-the-counter herbal therapies have further complicated the debate over what is the best therapeutic approach in patients with dyspepsia.

Thus, to elucidate the substantial number of issues relating to the diagnosis and management of dyspepsia, we have created this monograph. We have gathered an internationally recognized panel of experts and have challenged each of them to put in perspective the specific questions that pertain to the day-to-day clinical management of patients with dyspepsia. In this era of managed health care and cost containment, we have asked these experts to structure their discussions around clinical outcomes and to use an evidence-based approach. Whenever possible, the most cost-effective strategies are emphasized.

Dyspepsia is intended to bridge the gap between the exhaustive medical literature and the clinical decision-making involved in "the art of medicine." Our hope is that physicians will find that this pragmatic approach meets their needs in addressing common clinical questions and helps them to optimize clinical outcomes for their patients.

To our esteemed colleagues and contributors, we extend our thanks. You have exceeded our highest expectations and have provided all physicians with a powerful tool for examining more closely a very common yet complicated clinical dilemma.

David A. Johnson, MD
Philip O. Katz, MD
Donald O. Castell, MD

REFERENCES

1. **Talley NJ, Zinsmeister AR, Schleck CD, Melton LJ III.** Dyspepsia and dyspepsia subgroups: a population-based study. *Gastroenterology.* 1992;102:1259–68.

2. **Fisher RS, Parkman HP.** Management of nonulcer dyspepsia. *N Engl J Med.* 1998;339:1376–81.

3. **Reubin RJ, Cascade EF, Barker RC, et al.** Management of dyspepsia: a decision analysis. *Am J Manag Care.* 1996;2:647–55.

4. **McQuade KR.** Evolving approach to cyspepsia and nonulcer dyspepsia. *Gastrointest Dis Today.* 1997;6:1–9.

1

The Spectrum of Dyspepsia: Epidemiology, Etiology, and Natural History

Darryl Mackender, MB, BS(Syd), MPH

Nicholas J. Talley, MD, PhD

Dyspepsia is a common but poorly defined symptom complex occurring in the upper gastrointestinal tract and is a frequently seen presenting symptom in primary care and gastrointestinal practice. Dyspepsia can be a manifestation of varied and, in some cases, serious diseases; however, in approximately 50% of patients, no organic cause for dyspeptic symptoms is found after a thorough investigation. When this occurs, the symptoms are considered to be functional (or nonulcer) dyspepsia, a condition whose underlying pathophysiology may be protean and is poorly understood. There are many possible and, at times, costly investigations that may be used in the investigation of dyspepsia, although clearly these cannot be applied to all cases, given the common prevalence of these symptoms and the minimal yield from exhaustive investigations in most cases. Furthermore, because of the uncertainty surrounding the definition, pathogenesis, and relationship between symptom resolution and treatment, the optimal management strategy has long been controversial. For these reasons, various algorithms have been developed, recommending different treatment and investigative approaches that are based on patient characteristics and, more recently, *Helicobacter pylori* infection. In understanding the usefulness and cost effectiveness of these approaches, it is essential to examine the epidemiology and natural history of uninvestigated dyspepsia (i.e., dyspepsia for which no work-up has been undertaken) in the context of the changing epidemiology and natural history of the common underlying organic diseases that cause dyspepsia. Patients with uninvestigated dyspepsia may have any of the organic diseases associated with dyspepsia (Table 1.1), but most will have a final diagnosis of functional (or nonulcer) dyspepsia.

Definition of Dyspepsia

The definition of dyspepsia has changed over time, and many disparate definitions have been proposed over the last 25 years. The word *dyspepsia* can mean many different things to physicians, and patients usually have no idea what the word means. Dyspepsia is generally understood to be a symptom complex of the proximal alimentary tract and, in particular, the gastroduodenal region. This necessarily connotes an interpretation by the physician that symptoms arise from the upper gastrointestinal tract.

Although there have been many definitions proposed, the most widely accepted and authoritative definition is the Rome criteria (1,2) (recently revised), which define dyspepsia as chronic or recurrent pain or discomfort centered in the upper abdomen. The word *discomfort* refers to a subjective negative feeling that may be characterized by or associated with a number of painless symptoms, including upper abdominal fullness, early satiety, bloating, or nausea.

Based on 24-hour esophageal pH testing, there is a growing consensus that patients with a history of typical heartburn as the predominant symptom have symptomatic gastroesophageal reflux disease (GERD) until proven otherwise (3). There is reasonably good evidence that predominant heartburn is highly specific for GERD (3–5). Hence, the positive predictive value for predominant heartburn has been estimated to be between 59% and 81% in countries in which GERD is common (4,5).

Table 1.1   Organic Diseases Associated with Dyspepsia

- Peptic ulcer disease (duodenal and gastric ulcers)
- Cholelithiasis
- Gastroesophageal reflux disease
- Gastroparesis (motility disorder)
- Gastric cancer
- Pancreatic disease

Typical biliary colic with prolonged severe bouts of epigastric or right upper-quadrant pain usually is not considered to be part of the dyspeptic symptom complex (2). However, atypical presentations of biliary pathology (e.g., biliary dyskinesia) may result in symptoms that are indistinguishable from dyspepsia.

Epidemiology and Natural History of Dyspepsia

Dyspepsia is a remarkably common symptom complex. Approximately one in four persons in the community in the United States and Europe suffer with dyspepsia annually; however, only one quarter seek medical care (6). The point-prevalence rate of dyspepsia varies from 25% to 40%, although the higher rates seem to be explained by the inclusion of subjects with typical GERD (7). It has been estimated that approximately two thirds of the population has had dyspepsia at some time in their lives (8). The incidence of dyspepsia has been estimated to vary between 1% and 8% annually in the community; however, based on studies excluding relapsing patients, the incidence is most likely at the lower end of this range (9). Many patients present with mild symptoms of short duration (10). Approximately 30% of people with dyspeptic symptoms become asymptomatic over time, but approximately the same number of people who lose their symptoms experience a new onset of dyspepsia (9,11).

Dyspepsia accounts for 2% to 6% of primary care consultations and up to 40% of outpatient referrals to gastroenterologists (12–14). Dyspepsia may be an early symptom of a serious illness, such as peptic ulceration or gastric carcinoma. Even more importantly, dyspepsia has a considerable effect on individual suffering, medical workload, and financial burden. When considering the management of dyspepsia, it is important to take into account health care–seeking predictors and quality-of-life measures (especially the reassurance value of various strategies). In Europe, the vast majority of patients are managed by a primary care physician, with referral rates at first consultation for specialist care or investigations of 4% to 17% (13,14). Similar data are not available in the United States, but the rates are likely to vary across different parts of the country because of the wide array of health care choices. Decisions about referral or further investigation often seem as much a function of intuition as they are of clinical evidence. In developing a rational management approach, it is helpful to look at the changing epidemiology of underlying organic diseases. Indeed, patient age, racial background, geographic area, underlying *H. pylori* prevalence, and the relative epidemiology of particular organic diseases will alter the cost effectiveness of various options. It is also important to remember that the current epidemiology of dyspepsia is changing over time, due to both a falling *H. pylori* prevalence in certain populations (e.g., white U.S. citizens) and a waxing and waning in the prevalence of organic diseases. A particular management algorithm that is clinically useful and cost effective today may not be effective at all in 5 or 10 years.

Etiology of Dyspepsia

In addition to the major organic disorders shown in Table 1.1, a variety of other disorders may cause dyspepsia. These include medication-induced symptoms, endocrine or metabolic disturbances, pancreaticobiliary diseases, and luminal gastrointestinal disorders.

The sampling frame significantly influences the rate of detecting endoscopic findings in individuals with dyspepsia, and the rate in referred patients is likely to be different from that of the general population. In two population-based endoscopic studies among dyspepsia patients in Norway, only 9% of patients had a peptic ulcer and only 14% had esophagitis (15,16). Numerous other studies have demonstrated that peptic ulcer disease, reflux esophagitis, and cancer account for only a minority of dyspepsia cases. The remainder have either minor abnormalities of uncertain significance or an entirely normal endoscopy and are labeled as having functional (or nonulcer) dyspepsia. Regardless of definitions and methodology, it is clear that a substantial proportion of patients with dyspepsia (between 50%–70%) have no detectable organic disease.

Symptom Subgroups in Functional Dyspepsia

Because at least half of the individuals with dyspepsia have a negative diagnostic work-up, efforts have been made to identify clinical factors that are associated with the presence of organic disease.

Because many dyspepsia patients usually have multiple symptoms, it was proposed in 1988 that dyspepsia could be divided into subgroups (17). Specific groups of symptoms were labeled by consensus in the initial Rome definition of functional dyspepsia as either "ulcer-like" or "dysmotility-like" dyspepsia. "Reflux-like" dyspepsia was considered synonymous with symptomatic reflux disease (1). The use of symptom subgroups, however, has been disappointing, mostly because of the extensive overlap of the subgroups based on symptom groupings and because a substantial proportion of patients could not be classified using this approach at all (unspecified dyspepsia) (2). More importantly, the symptom subgroups have not been particularly useful in identifying relevant disease or response to treatment.

The most recent Rome II consensus suggests that the subgroup classification should be based on the predominant or most bothersome single symptom identified by the patient, rather than by clusters of complaints (2). Among patients with functional dyspepsia, those who have ulcer-like dyspepsia (in which epigastric *pain* is the predominant complaint) are more likely to benefit from potent antisecretory therapy than those who have dysmotility-like dyspepsia (in which epigastric *discomfort* [e.g., bloating, fullness, early satiety, nausea] is the predominant complaint) (18). This approach, however, still requires careful validation.

Alarm Features That Identify Structural Disease

In 1985, the American College of Physicians (ACP) published guidelines for the management of dyspepsia based on a review of the literature (19). It was suggested that a trial of therapy was initially appropriate in most patients. The guidelines emphasized the need to search clinically for alarm features that would indicate a more serious diagnosis.

Age has been applied as a means of identifying patients at higher risk of having structural disease. Traditionally, an age of over 45 years has been used since publication of the ACP guidelines; however, more recently, data from the United Kingdom suggest that an age of over 55 years may be a more appropriate threshold because of the changing epidemiology of peptic ulcer disease and gastric cancer (20).

Other alarm features that are typically applied include weight loss, vomiting, progressive dysphagia, odynophagia, bleeding, anemia, jaundice, abdominal mass, and lymphadenopathy.

Because there are few available studies in the literature, the value of these alarm symptoms and signs for identifying those at higher risk of structural disease is based largely on clinical judgment. Some general observations also can be made based on three studies that evaluated unintentional weight loss in patients without dyspepsia (21–23). The causes most frequently found were cancer, psychiatric disease, and gastrointestinal disease. Although gastrointestinal disorders were common, the specific diagnoses varied markedly among the studies, ranging from malabsorption, inflammatory bowel disease, and peptic ulcer disease to esophageal dysmotility and hepatitis. However, the absence of alarm symptoms in young dyspeptic patients presenting for endoscopy seems to be a reasonably reliable indicator that gastrointestinal malignancy is not present (24).

Major Organic Diseases Underlying Dyspepsia

Peptic Ulceration, Gastritis, and Duodenitis
Peptic ulcer disease, either gastric or duodenal, is one of the most common organic causes of dyspepsia. The definition of peptic ulceration and its distinction from erosions in most studies is based on the depth of mucosal

penetration (25). There is general consensus that endoscopy is superior to barium radiography in evaluating the esophagus, stomach, and duodenum (10,26,27). Nevertheless, current endoscopic diagnosis is inaccurate for depth and relies on the appearance of slough in an ulcer base (which may be poorly seen with hemorrhage) or more consistently is based on size (usually with erosion <5 mm and ulcer ≥5 mm [28]). When fiber-optic endoscopy is not available, interpretation of historical changes and understanding the epidemiology of peptic ulcer disease is hampered by the limitations of barium radiography of the upper gastrointestinal tract.

Predicting previous peptic ulceration is difficult. A carefully taken medical history of previous peptic ulceration is usually inaccurate. In a thorough Scandinavian population study of peptic ulcer prevalence, a false-positive reporting rate of 15% to 20% and a false-negative reporting rate of 0.2% to 1.3% was observed based on a careful review of all medical records (15). In same study, a point-prevalence rate of 3.2% for deformed duodenal bulbs in healthy controls (especially in women) suggested that either duodenal ulcer disease was often either asymptomatic or underdiagnosed in women. There are limited other data on the epidemiology of deformed duodenal bulbs and on the relevance of this finding in the investigation of dyspepsia. Similarly, there is little information on the usefulness of diagnostic sensitivity and specificity of gastric ulcer scars in predicting past or future peptic ulceration. Gastric ulcer scars are difficult to see on conventional endoscopy (29).

Gastritis is inflammation of the gastric mucosa and, hence, a pathologic rather than clinical endoscopic or radiologic diagnosis. Physicians and patients often use the term *gastritis* when more accurate terms would be *dyspepsia* or *heartburn*. Endoscopists often use the term gastritis as a synonym for erythema or friability of the mucosa or "submucosal hemorrhage" (it is also impossible to predict depth of hemorrhage at endoscopy) (30). Multiple studies have shown that gastritis cannot be diagnosed on the basis of the endoscopic appearance of the gastric mucosa (30). Identifying a causal link between dyspepsia and histologic gastritis has been difficult (31,32). Likewise, duodenitis should be a histologic diagnosis, although the appearances of gastric metaplasia at endoscopy are characteristic. It is likely, however, that these endoscopic changes may be subtle or patchy and easily missed, and the prevalence of gastric metaplasia and duodenitis may be much higher if biopsies were performed more often. There is general agreement that, unlike gastritis and gastric ulceration, a more reliable correlation exists between significant erosive duodenitis and true duodenal ulceration (33). It is our belief that a patient with significant duodenitis and gastric metaplasia should be treated as having a duodenal ulcer diathesis and considered at high risk for current or future duodenal ulceration.

Gastroesophageal Reflux Disease

The spectrum of GERD ranges from asymptomatic physiologic events in relation to meals to a relapsing, severe, incapacitating, and even life-threatening disease complicated by ulcerative inflammation and strictures of the esophagus. The natural history of GERD is not well known. Only a few studies have focused on the natural history of typical GERD, with or without endoscopic esophagitis. In a study by Pace and coworkers (34), patients with GERD were followed for 6 months, during which time 15% of the patients developed new endoscopic esophagitis despite symptomatic treatment. Another study of a larger population of patients found that nearly half of the patients had only isolated episodes of esophagitis, whereas the other half had chronic disease (35). Although this study had limitations, it implied that there is a subgroup of patients who have only isolated episodes of symptomatic reflux with or without esophagitis, whereas in most patients the disease is chronic.

There is no accepted and precise definition of GERD nor is there a gold standard. The symptoms can be variable, even absent. Although diagnostic procedures have improved considerably during the past 10 years, there is still some doubt as to what the gold standard should be—symptoms, endoscopic appearance, results of 24-hour esophageal pH monitoring, or therapeutic response to proton-pump inhibitors.

Heartburn is well recognized as the predominant symptom of GERD, and acid regurgitation is also thought to be relatively specific for predicting reflux disease (1). An assessment of these symptoms in a population-based setting by questionnaire has been shown to correlate well with results from primary care physician assessments and gastroenterologist interviews (36).

The macroscopic appearance of endoscopic esophagitis can range from subtle alterations in mucosal erythema, edema, and mucosal friability to unequivocal signs of severe esophagitis with circumferential and confluent erosions and ulceration. Many classifications of these appearances are based, albeit loosely, on the original proposal of Savary and Miller (37). However, there is no general agreement on what constitutes the minimum recognizable indicator of reflux esophagitis. Because the definitions of endoscopic esophagitis are so disparate, it is difficult to determine and compare the outcomes of many studies.

Bytzer and coworkers (38) reported good agreement between three endoscopists for moderate to severe esophagitis; however, there was poor agreement for mild esophagitis, providing further support for the lack of specificity of "soft signs," such as diffuse erythema, edema, congestion, mucosal friability, and isolated areas of erythema not covered by fibrin. A more recent classification system for endoscopic esophagitis (the Los Angeles system) relies on visible mucosal breaks and their extent and seems to have high diagnostic value and good interobserver validity even at the milder grades of esophagitis (39). Various indices of so-called "pathological acid reflux" on 24-hour esophageal pH studies have been chosen, most typically the time with pH < 4, and total acid exposure time. A proportion (20%) of patients with no endoscopic esophagitis and dyspepsia (heartburn not predominant) has pathological acid reflux by these criteria (40), although the implications for the management of dyspepsia are unclear. More recently, the correlation between patient-triggered symptom markers and reflux episodes on 24-hour pH study (symptom index [SI]) has been proposed as another index of true reflux disease in the absence of pathological acid reflux (41).

A brief trial of a standard or high-dose proton-pump inhibitor—initially used as a "diagnostic test" for discriminating between reflux and other causes of chest pain—has been suggested as a possible test for discriminating between reflux disease and dyspepsia (including functional dyspepsia) (18,42,43). The clinical use of this approach (and, in particular, the effectiveness in selecting patients for endoscopy and the correlation with endoscopic esophagitis or pH testing) awaits prospective validation. (*See* Chapter 3 for more information on other diagnostic tests for GERD.)

Carcinomas of the Upper Gastrointestinal Tract

The histologic and clinical distinction between carcinomas of the proximal esophagus (squamous cell carcinomas) and of the distal esophagus (adenocarcinomas) is clear cut and likely has not changed over the years. An undisputed true increase in esophageal adenocarcinoma has been seen despite some change due to improved specification of diagnosis with increasing use of endoscopy (44). Similarly, the rates of Barrett's esophagus (and the more recently described short-segment Barrett's esophagus) probably have been altered substantially with the increased use of endoscopy (45). Any apparent increase in the prevalence of Barrett's esophagus is likely due to increased diagnosis, given that studies in unselected autopsies have suggested the autopsy prevalence of Barrett's is 20-fold higher than in clinically diagnosed cases (45).

Gastroparesis

Patients with gastroparesis usually present with recurrent, disabling, and severe nausea and vomiting, both with liquids and solids. Vomiting of undigested food may make differentiation from gastric outlet obstruction difficult. Weight loss and malnutrition are the rule. Gastroparesis is usually seen in patients with underlying systemic sclerosis, chronic infectional pseudo-obstruction, acute or chronic renal failure (associated with uremia), diabetes mellitus (with autonomic neuropathy), and rarely postviral syndrome; however, many cases are not associated with these systemic disorders and are termed *idiopathic*. Although these patients also may have dyspepsia, confusion with functional dyspepsia is unlikely, and the approach to diagnosis is different (*see* Chapter 5).

Historical Epidemiology

Interpreting historical changes in disease patterns is complicated by changing information sources, alterations in diagnostic labels, cohort effects, and the confounding effect of changes in the age distribution of populations. Despite these limitations, there is confidence that some broad changes in the historical epidemiology of dyspepsia and underlying organic diseases have occurred. These changes have had a significant effect on the usefulness and cost effectiveness of various management algorithms.

Dyspepsia

Despite some changes in definition, it seems that the overall prevalence of dyspepsia is little different now than it was when early surveys of U.K. communities found the prevalence to be 30% in 1951 (46) and 25% in 1968 (47). There has been increasing awareness of atypical presentations, such as the emergence of noncardiac chest pain and its relationship to GERD and the concurrence of irritable bowel symptoms and functional dyspepsia. However, overall, the epidemiologic pattern seems to have remained the same. Dyspepsia occurs with similar frequency in men and women, increases in prevalence with advancing age, and remains unexplained or idiopathic (nonulcer or functional) in most patients despite exhaustive diagnostic work-ups and some changes in the frequency of underlying organic diseases. However, there is evidence that a significant epidemiologic change has taken place over the years in the organic diseases that cause dyspepsia. This will have an effect on the usefulness of various management algorithms employed now and in the future.

Peptic Ulcer Disease

The history of uncomplicated ulcers is partially obscured by changes in diagnostic practices and by the selection of patients who are admitted to a hospital or examined at autopsy. Studies from England were the first to report that mortality and hospital admissions rates for peptic ulceration were declining (48). However, it has been estimated that the incidence of uncomplicated duodenal and gastric ulcers has decreased over the past 30 years in the United States by approximately 70% and 50%, respectively, based on rates of ulcer surgery, hospital admissions, mortality, and physician visits (49) (Fig. 1.1).

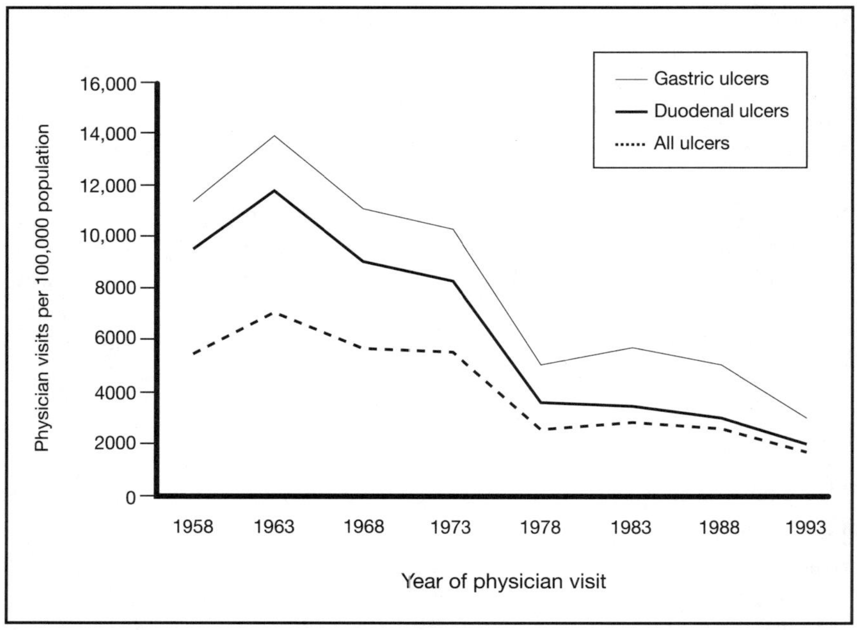

Figure 1.1   Time trends of physicians visits for peptic ulcer from 1958 to 1993. (Data from El-Serag HB, Sonnenberg A. Opposing time trends of peptic ulcer and reflux disease. *Gut.* 1998;43:327–33.)

The incidence of acute perforations is one of the most useful and robust indicators of historical change, and it can be reconstructed from available records in several countries. In 1940, Jennings (48) analyzed mortality from peptic ulcer perforations in London hospitals from the previous century. He described three different clinical syndromes that dominated at different periods. In the early 19th century, the prevailing syndrome of perforations was gastric ulceration near the cardia seen among young women. By the late 19th century, the syndrome not only involved gastric ulcer perforations but also juxtapyloric and chronic perforations seen in older men and women. In the early 20th century, duodenal ulcer perforations were seen especially in young men and, later, in middle-aged men. Using cohort analysis (50,51) and keeping in mind the historical epidemiology of *H. pylori,* closer analysis of these data suggests that, in men, a regression of the wave of peptic ulcer began in the new generations of the higher social classes and occurred first with gastric ulceration followed by duodenal ulceration, with a delay of 10 years (50,52).

Rates of duodenal ulcer bleeding have not decreased during the past 20 years, and gastric ulcer bleeding rates have increased more than twofold (53).

The increased incidence of bleeding ulcers, especially in elderly women, may be due to increased nonsteroidal anti-inflammatory drug (NSAID) use and possibly increased smoking among women during this period (16).

There is some suggestion that peptic ulcer perforation is less common than in previous decades, although this does not seem to be attributable solely to more effective treatment or to *H. pylori* eradication (54–56). Since the introduction of H_2-receptor antagonists (H2RAs) in 1978, the incidence of surgery for peptic ulcer disease has decreased markedly, although this is a trend that has been documented since the early 1960s (57,58). So, although the disappearance of *H. pylori* in Western populations (as described below) likely has reduced the incidence of perforated peptic ulcer disease in parallel with a reduction in overall ulcer prevalence, there may be other contributing factors.

Epidemiology of *Helicobacter pylori* Infection

Spiral gastric bacteria have been identified in the human stomach since 1906 (59). In 1983, Warren and Marshall (60) isolated *H. pylori* from gastric specimens and launched a revolution, not only in our thinking of acid-peptic diseases but also in the management of dyspepsia. Indeed, without the knowledge of *H. pylori*'s principal role in causing some of the traditional organic diseases in dyspepsia, much of the discussion about effective management algorithms for uninvestigated dyspepsia would not have occurred.

To understand the possible role for noninvasive testing for *H. pylori* infection and the implications of *H. pylori* diagnosis at the time of endoscopy, knowledge of local geographical prevalence, background ethnic and socioeconomic determinants, and temporal changes in *H. pylori* epidemiology is required. Because our understanding of the implications of naturally occurring and treatment-related changes in the prevalence of *H. pylori* is limited, recommendations for future management of dyspepsia may need to be reviewed as *H. pylori* becomes a less prevalent infection.

Geographic Epidemiology

The seroprevalence of *H. pylori* infection has been verified in most countries around the world. In developing nations, the infection is probably acquired early in life (childhood or even infancy); hence, most individuals are infected by early adulthood (61). In developed countries, a progressive increase in the rate of *H. pylori* infection is associated with increasing age, with the prevalence being most common (approximately 40%–60%) in the elderly but rare in children (52). Longitudinal studies have suggested that this distribution is due chiefly to an age-cohort phenomenon (51), which is what occurs when an infection was much more common in the children of earlier generations who then carried their infection through life. Low socioeconomic status in childhood is considered to be the major risk factor for *H. pylori* infection, although it is unclear why low socioeconomic status in childhood confers a greater risk (52). Although traditional correlates of low socioeconomic status (e.g., smoking, drinking alcohol) have not been shown to affect the prevalence of *H. pylori* in a population (62), other determinants (e.g., household crowding, bed sharing, lack of hot water, number of siblings [52,62,63]) *are* associated with a high risk of *H. pylori* infection, suggesting a close-contact, person-to-person spread via oral-oral or fecal-oral routes.

The limited available data suggest the importance of considering the geographic and socioeconomic context of a patient's childhood when estimating his or her likely background *H. pylori* prevalence; the usefulness of various management algorithms may be affected.

Temporal Epidemiology

Indirect evidence, chiefly found in developed countries, suggests a rapidly falling risk of childhood and early adulthood *H. pylori* infection for those born after 1950. This abrupt change has been attributed euphemistically to "improved social conditions." Banatvala and coworkers (51) showed a progressive decrease in the rate of infection in each cohort based on sera stored from 1969, 1979, and 1989. Clearly, this decrease began long before the discovery of *H. pylori* and its role in acid-peptic disease, but it is likely that that the population prevalence will continue to fall even more rapidly with the increasing enthusiasm for *H. pylori* eradication that is currently being adopted.

With the now well-established link between persistent *H. pylori* infection and the risk of duodenal and non-NSAID gastric ulceration (63), it is tempting simply to superimpose the epidemiology of peptic ulcer disease on the limited knowledge we have of the epidemiology of *H. pylori* infection. Logically, the incidence of *H. pylori*-associated ulcer disease will decline gradually with the decreasing rates of *H. pylori* infection, and then either NSAID-associated ulcers or non-NSAID, non-*H. pylori* ulcers will become more common than *H. pylori*-associated ulcers. A recent study of a multiracial population in greater Rochester, New York, suggested that 30% of duodenal ulcer patients were *H. pylori* negative on urease test and antral histology (non-NSAID use was confirmed by serum salicylate levels) (64). When analyzed by racial background, 50% of non-NSAID duodenal ulcers in whites were *H. pylori* negative compared with 15% in nonwhites (i.e., blacks, Hispanics, and Asians). In a community-based gastroenterology practice in Orlando, Florida, only 27% of patients with non–NSAID-associated duodenal ulcers tested positive for *H. pylori* infection (65), and a smaller retrospective study from Australia found that only 55% of patients with duodenal ulcers tested positive for *H. pylori* (66).

The likely increase in the prevalence of non–*H. pylori*-associated gastric and duodenal ulcer disease (in conjunction with newer, possibly less ulcerogenic Cox-2–specific NSAIDs) will have a significant effect on the future efficacy of management approaches for uninvestigated dyspepsia. The variations on the *H. pylori* "test and treat" or "test and scope" strategies will be cost effective and clinically useful only in the presence of a significant background prevalence of *H. pylori* infection and *H. pylori*-associated diseases.

Epidemiology of Gastroesophageal Reflux Disease, Barrett's Esophagus, and Gastrointestinal Malignancy

The frequency of heartburn, the predominant symptom of GERD, has not changed in the past two decades (67). The evaluation of esophagitis epidemiology over this period has been hampered by inadequate diagnostic tools and disparate definitions. Previous estimates of GERD have been based on the reflux of barium on upper gastrointestinal barium radiography and are, therefore, inaccurate due to poor correlation with endoscopic esophagitis or pathological acid reflux (68). In 1969, a population-based study in Scotland found that only 47% of patients with severe esophagitis detected by rigid esophagogastroscopy demonstrated barium reflux (69). Because Barrett's esophagus cannot be diagnosed with barium radiography, the historical epidemiology of Barrett's esophagus cannot be assessed for the time period before endoscopy was in widespread use.

Based on all routine upper gastrointestinal barium studies that had been carried out in northeastern Scotland, Brunnen and coworkers (69) estimated in 1969 the prevalence of GERD (by barium radiography) to be 86 per 100,000 per year and the prevalence of severe esophagitis (by rigid esophagogastroscopy) to be 4.5 per 100,000 per year. In 1993, a similar study based on endoscopic reports from a defined area in Sweden suggested a similar incidence of GERD, finding esophagitis in 120 per 100,000 per year and complicated esophagitis in 5.6 per 100,000 per year (70). However, recent data from hospitalization and mortality data in Veterans Affairs patients in the United States suggest that between 1970 and 1995 hospitalization and death rates for erosive esophagitis have been increasing (44). Although this, in part, may represent more widespread use of endoscopy and better grading of esophagitis, there also may be a recent change in the epidemiology of GERD.

In light of the undisputed exponential rise in adenocarcinoma of the esophagus and gastric cardia (chiefly among white men [20,71]) and the known falling prevalence of *H. pylori*, it has been proposed that, with the eradication of *H. pylori*, there will be an increased incidence of GERD, Barrett's esophagus, and subsequent adenocarcinoma of the esophagus. However, the epidemiologic link between these diseases is not so easily deduced.

Little evidence exists to support the contention that there is an increased incidence of Barrett's esophagus, and there is evidence suggesting that certain strains of *H. pylori* actually may protect against esophagitis. Recent reports from Germany suggest that up to 26% of duodenal ulcer patients who had undergone successful *H. pylori* eradication developed reflux esophagitis compared with 13% of duodenal ulcer patients who were still infected (72). However, large studies from Europe (73) and Australia (74) found no clear-cut increase in the frequency of heartburn or of reflux esophagitis after *H. pylori* eradication. It has been suggested that CagA-positive strains of *H. pylori* are protective for esophagitis (10). In regions of the world where infection rates with CagA-positive strains of *H. pylori* are high (e.g., China, Japan) (75), the incidence of endoscopically proven esophagitis is low (76,77). The prevalence of reflux symptoms among hospital outpatients (78), pregnant women (79), and the general population (76) seems to be much lower in multiracial populations in the East (Fig. 1.2). Likewise, the prevalence of endoscopic esophagitis is lower in Asia (76,77). (It is interesting in this context to note that, to date, the word *heartburn* has no di-

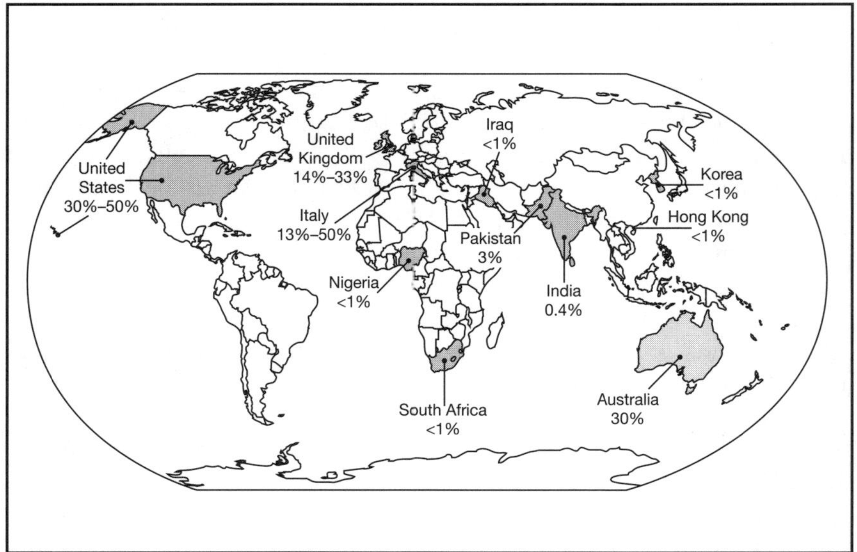

Figure 1.2   Percent prevalence of reflux disease/hiatal hernia in selected countries.

rect Chinese, Malaysian, or Indian translation.) Although this difference may be attributable to certain strains of *H. pylori* common in Asia and less common in the West (80), there is also some suggestion that Asian patients may have reduced esophageal mucosal acid sensitivity, lesser degrees of pathological reflux, and/or greater mucosal acid resistance than their Western counterparts (81). Eradication of *H. pylori* in these areas may predict the worsening of GERD more reliably. In contrast, however, the eradication of *H. pylori* may have little effect on GERD in regions of the world where the prevalence of *H. pylori* is lower and is colonized primarily by CagA-negative strains, such as in the United States, Europe, and Australia (81).

Epidemiology of Upper Gastrointestinal Malignancy

There is a well-established downward trend in the incidence of gastric cancer worldwide. From the late 1970s to 1990s, the incidence of adenocarcinoma of the distal esophagus and gastric cardia increased more rapidly than any other cancer in the United States (40) (Figs. 1.3 and 1.4), where an estimated 25,000 people die of these cancers every year (82).

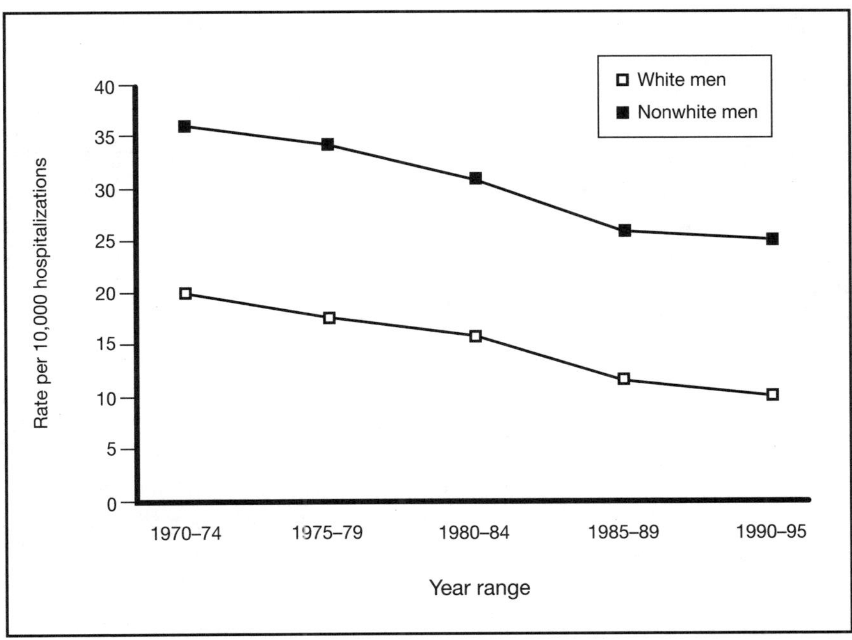

Figure 1.3   Time trends of hospitalization for cancer of the gastric corpus and antrum. (Data from El-Serag HB, Sonnenberg A. Opposing time trends of peptic ulcer and reflux disease. *Gut.* 1998;43:327–33.)

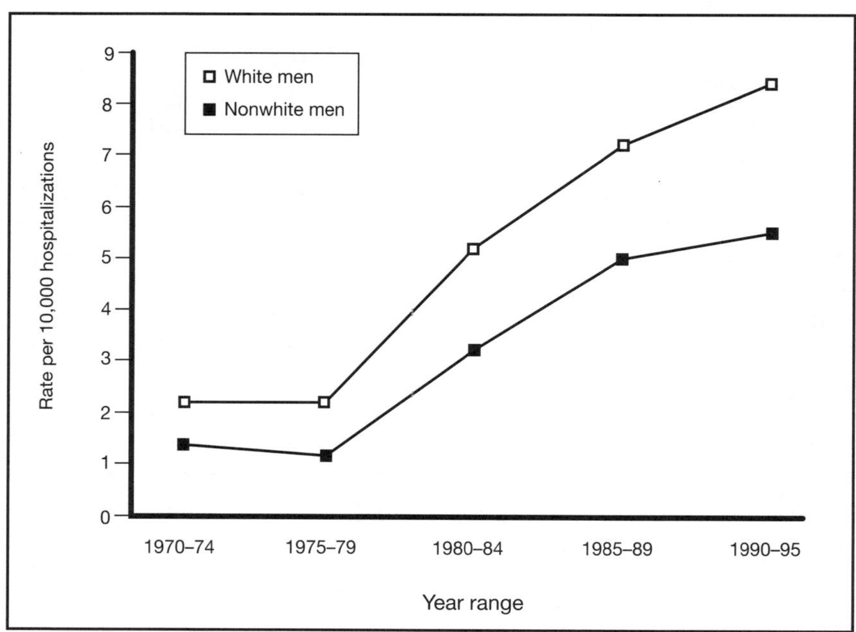

Figure 1.4   Time trends of hospitalization rates for cancer of the gastric cardia. (Data from El-Serag HB, Sonnenberg A. Opposing time trends of peptic ulcer and reflux disease. *Gut.* 1998;43:327–33.)

The presence of gastric cancer is rare in individuals younger than 45 years of age, whereas its incidence rapidly increases thereafter in Western nations. Some countries in Asia and the Pacific islands, however, have an age-specific incidence of gastric cancer that begins to rise after the age of 35 years (83); therefore, a lower age threshold in immigrants from these regions may be appropriate.

Self-Care

As mentioned earlier in this chapter, approximately one in four U.S. citizens in the community suffers with dyspepsia; however, only one quarter of these seek medical care. Self-care is obviously important. Studies have shown that 20% of the general population are self-medicating for symptoms of GERD and heartburn. In a random population in Minneapolis, 22% (28% of whom had dyspepsia without GERD, 67% with GERD) reported using over-the-counter (OTC) H2RAs in the past year; 15.5% of these did so at least monthly, 93% did so in conjunction with at least one other medication, but only 15% achieved complete relief (84). The availability of more effective OTC-H2RA treatment initially created expectations for decreased medical expenditures by decreasing physician visits, but these expectations have not been fulfilled (85).

Influence of the Epidemiology of Dyspepsia on Various Management Options

Determining the optimal management strategy has long been a matter of controversy for several reasons. Because the exact cause of dyspepsia is difficult to identify, seemingly appropriate treatments may not result in symptom resolution. The cost effectiveness of management approaches is a matter of debate, because "avoiding" costly diagnostic tests is pitted against less expensive empirical trials that may or may not yield results that are helpful in guiding therapy. Considering the epidemiology of the disorders, therefore, is another way of clarifying the difficult matter of assessing management algorithms.

Symptom Resolution

Symptoms drive health care expenditure. In assessing various management algorithms for uninvestigated dyspepsia, it is important to realize that there is not always a good correlation between 1) the treatment and resolution of endoscopic lesions (ulcers or esophagitis) and 2) the complete resolution of symptoms. Even in early trials of *H. pylori* eradication in duodenal ulcer patients, 7-year follow-up showed recurrent symptoms in 42% of patients who remained *H. pylori* positive and in 22% of patients who had their *H. pylori* eradicated (86). If applied to some management algorithms, a high failure rate for a "test and treat" strategy would have significant effects on costs—especially if these "failures" continue with consultation, investigation, and care.

There is also a significant background of asymptomatic organic disease in patients with dyspepsia. Peptic ulcer disease is a chronic disease characterized by frequent relapses in the absence of *H. pylori* eradication, followed by varying periods without dyspeptic symptoms. Other studies have reported that after 4 to 8 years of follow-up, up to 47% of gastric ulcer recurrences may again be asymptomatic (87). There is also no guarantee that a normal endoscopy precludes the future development of organic disease. Two recent large trials of *H. pylori* eradication in functional dyspepsia both showed a 5% risk of developing peptic ulceration over 12 months (31,32), and others have observed higher rates (88). Clearly, this apparent crossover from functional dyspepsia to organic disease will alter the usefulness and cost effectiveness of various management algorithms.

Prompt Endoscopy

There is evidence that selected patients who are referred for and receive prompt endoscopy have a better outcome than those who are prescribed empirical H2RAs. In a randomized trial, Bytzer and coworkers (89) found that prompt endoscopy was followed by significantly greater symptom improvement and satisfaction scores at 4 weeks compared with those randomized to empirical H2RAs. Furthermore, two thirds of patients on empirical therapy eventually underwent endoscopy during the 12-month follow-up. Other studies have shown that, after endoscopy, dyspepsia patients seem to be more reassured and require fewer prescriptions (90,91); however, not all studies agree (92). Moreover, it is likely that endoscopy services would be overwhelmed if all patients with dyspepsia who present for care were recommended for an endoscopic procedure.

With the changing epidemiology of underlying organic disease in dyspepsia, it is interesting to note that a recent study suggested that the endoscopic findings in a series of patients with GERD symptoms did not alter management (93). Other studies document significant alterations in management based on endoscopic findings in reflux esophagitis, with treatment intensifying in 74% of those with severe esophagitis and decreasing in 65% of those with negative endoscopic findings (94). It may be that a high-dose trial of proton-pump inhibitors is as useful a discriminating test for reflux disease as endoscopy, although this approach still awaits careful prospective validation.

Helicobacter pylori "Test and Treat" Strategy

The rationale behind testing for *H. pylori* in patients with dyspepsia is to help identify those with peptic ulcer disease (or gastric cancer) who require appropriate management. In Scotland, McColl and coworkers (95) have shown that, among patients presenting to their physician with dyspepsia who had a positive urea breath test, 40% had duodenal ulcer, 13% had gastric ulcer, 1% had a deformed duodenum, 2% had erosive duodenitis, and 12% had esophagitis. This was in striking contrast to those patients who had a negative urea breath test—only 2% had duodenal ulcer, only 3% had gastric ulcer, and 17% had esophagitis (95).

Because anxiety and the fear of serious disease are factors that drive people with dyspepsia to seek health care, the issue of adequately reassuring patients must be addressed. There is some evidence that *H. pylori* testing, if negative, is reassuring. When *H. pylori* testing is positive, performing subsequent endoscopy seems to be equally reassuring (96). However, recent studies of the reassurance value of the "test and treat" strategy are less encouraging (97).

Eradicating *H. pylori* infection does not relieve the symptoms in all patients with peptic ulcer disease (86), and it is thought that some patients may develop new reflux symptoms (72). Moreover, in most cases, the symptoms in functional dyspepsia will not be relieved by *H. pylori* eradication (31,32). Clearly, this will have an effect on the usefulness of a "test and treat" strategy if these patients with new or persistent symptoms still require investigation. Furthermore, one must consider that the *H. pylori* "test and treat" strategy requires a moderate to high prevalence of *H. pylori* colonization and *H. pylori*-associated ulcer disease to be cost effective.

Conclusions

As a presenting problem to primary care practitioners, dyspepsia is no less common now than it was two decades ago, despite the release of OTC H2RAs and a decreasing prevalence of *H. pylori*. However, the epidemiology of possible underlying organic diseases has changed significantly. Most patients with dyspepsia have no significant abnormality on endoscopy, and their symptoms seem to fluctuate over time for unclear reasons, with some patients having prolonged symptom-free periods. With the passage of time, the prevalence of *H. pylori*-associated organic diseases (e.g., peptic ulcer disease, gastric cancer) will become increasingly less common. A greater proportion of underlying organic disease will be NSAID-associated ulcers or non-NSAID, non-*H. pylori* ulcers. It is also likely that reflux esophagitis and esophageal adenocarcinoma will become more common. This will have a significant influence on the clinical usefulness and cost effectiveness of the approaches to investigating and managing dyspepsia.

Thus, although the overall prevalence of organic diseases underlying dyspepsia may be no different, the implications of detecting underlying GERD (usually without esophagitis) are different from those of recurrent peptic ulcer disease (which may cause death). The usefulness of endoscopy in the investigation of dyspepsia increasingly will rely on its reassurance value and its effect on quality of life and future consultations. Our understanding of the underlying pathophysiology of dyspepsia (most cases of which show no endoscopic abnormality) also has implications for targeting more effective treatments.

Key Points

- Dyspepsia is a common but poorly understood symptom complex defined as chronic or recurrent pain or discomfort centered in the upper abdomen.
- *Functional* or *nonulcer* dyspepsia refers to dyspeptic symptoms for which no organic cause is found.

- Approximately one in four persons in the United States and Europe has dyspepsia, accounting for 2% to 6% of primary care visits and for up to 40% of outpatient referrals to gastroenterologists.

- Dyspepsia may be caused by any of several underlying disorders, some of which may represent serious disease. Major underlying organic diseases include peptic ulcer disease, GERD, motility disorders, and gastric cancer.

- Over the past 30 years, the incidence of uncomplicated duodenal ulcer and gastric ulcer in the United States has decreased 70% and 50%, respectively. This may be attributed in part to a decrease in *H. pylori* infection resulting from improved socioeconomic conditions, the recent discovery of the role of *H. pylori* in peptic ulcer disease, and the consequent use of therapies aimed at eradicating *H. pylori*.

- With the decreased incidence of *H. pylori* infection, a greater proportion of the diseases underlying dyspepsia will include NSAID-associated ulcers, reflux esophagitis, and esophageal adenocarcinoma. This changing epidemiology will in turn alter the cost effectiveness of current management approaches.

REFERENCES

1. **Talley NJ, Colin-Jones D, Koch KL, et al.** Functional dyspepsia: a classification with guidelines for diagnosis and management. *Gastroenterol Int.* 1991;4:145–60.

2. **Talley NJ, Stanghellini V, Heading RC, et al.** Functional gastroduodenal disorders. *Gut.* 1999;45(Suppl2)1137–42.

3. **Dent J, Brun J, Fendrick AM, et al.** An evidence-based appraisal of reflux disease management: The Genval Workshop report. *Gut.* 1999;44:S1–16.

4. **Klauser AG, Schindlbeck NE, Muller-Lissner SA.** Symptoms in gastroesophageal reflux disease. *Lancet.* 1990;335:205–8.

5. **Johnsson F, Joelsson B, Gudmunsson K, Greiff L.** Symptoms and endoscopic findings in the diagnosis of gastroesophageal reflux disease. *Scand J Gastroenterol.* 1987;22:714–8.

6. **Klauser AG, Voderholzer WA, Knesewitsch PA, et al.** What is behind dyspepsia? *Dig Dis Sci.* 1993;38:147–54.

7. **Richter JE, Castell DO.** Gastroesophageal reflux: pathogenesis, diagnosis, and therapy. *Ann Intern Med.* 1982;97:93.

8. **Jones R, Lydeard S.** Prevalence of symptoms of dyspepsia in the community. *Lancet.* 1989;47–51.

9. **Talley NJ, Weaver AL, Zinsmeister AR, Melton LJ.** Onset and disappearance of gastrointestinal symptoms and functional gastrointestinal disorders. *Am J Epidemiol.* 1992;136:165.

10. **Dooley CP, Larson AW, Stace NH, et al.** Double-contrast barium meal and upper gastrointestinal endoscopy: a comparative study. *Ann Intern Med.* 1984;101:538–45.

11. **Meineche-Schmidt V, Christensen E.** Classification of dyspepsia: identification of independent symptom components in 7270 consecutive, unselected dyspepsia patients from general practice. *Scand J Gastroenterol.* 1998;33:1262–72.

12. **Knill-Jones RP.** Geographical differences in the prevalence of dyspepsia. *Scand J Gastroenterol.* 1991;26(Suppl 182):17.

13. **Warndorff DK, Knottnerus JA, Huijen LGJ, Starmans R.** How well do general practitioners manage dyspepsia? *J R Coll Gen Pract.* 1989;39:499–502.

14. **Heikkinen M, Pikkrainen P, Takala J, Julkunen R.** General practitioners' approach to dyspepsia: survey of consultation frequencies, treatment, and investigation. *Scand J Gastroenterol.* 1996;31:648–53.

15. **Bernerson B, Johnsen R, Straume B, et al.** Towards a true prevalence of peptic ulcer: the Sorreisa Gastrointestinal Disorder Study. *Gut.* 1990;31:989–92.

16. **Johnsen R, Bernerson B, Straume B, et al.** Prevalences of endoscopic and histological findings in subjects with and without dyspepsia. *BMJ.* 1991;302:749–52.

17. **Colin-Jones DG.** Management of dyspepsia: report of a working party. *Lancet.* 1988;1:576–9.

18. **Talley NJ, Axon A, Bytzer P, et al.** Management of uninvestigated and functional dyspepsia: a Working Party report for the World Congresses of Gastroenterology. *Aliment Pharmacol Ther.* 1999;19:1135–48.

19. **Health and Public Policy Committee, American College of Physicians.** Endoscopy in the evaluation of dyspepsia. *Ann Intern Med.* 1985;102:266–9.

20. **Pera M, Cameron AJ, Trastek VF, et al.** Increasing incidence of adenocarcinoma of the esophagus and esophagogastric junction.*Gastroenterology.* 1993;104:510–3.

21. **Martin KI, Sox HC, Krupp JR.** Involuntary weight loss: diagnostic and prognostic significance. *Ann Intern Med.* 1981;95:568.

22. **Rabinovitz M, Pitlik SD, Leifer M, et al.** Unintentional weight loss: a retrospective analysis of 154 cases. *Arch Intern Med.* 1986;146:186.

23. **Thompson MP, Morris LK.** Unexplained weight loss in the ambulatory elderly. *J Am Geriatr Soc.* 1991;39:497.

24. **Gillen D, McColl KE.** Does concern about missing malignancy justify endoscopy in uncomplicated dyspepsia in patients aged less than 55? *Am J Gastroenterol.* 1999;94:75–9.

25. **Borch K, Jansson L, Sjodahl R et al.** Hemorrhagic gastritis: incidence, etiological factors, and prognosis. *Acta Chir Scand.* 1987;154:211.

26. **Martin TR, Vennes JA, Silvis SE, Ansel HJ.** A comparison of upper gastrointestinal endoscopy and radiography. *J Clin Gastroenterol.* 1980;2:21–5.

27. **Shaw PC, van Romounde LK, Griffioen G, et al.** Peptic ulcer and gastric carcinoma: diagnosis with biphasic radiography compared with fibreoptic endoscopy. *Radiology.* 1987;163:39–42.

28. **Elta GH.** Approach to the patient with gross intestinal bleeding. In Yamada T, et al. (eds). *Textbook of Gastroenterology,* 2nd ed. Philadelphia: JB Lippincott; 1995:676.

29. **Sakaki N, Momma K, Egawa N, et al.** Preliminary clinical study on gastric ulcer scars and ulcer relapses after *Helicobacter pylori* eradication therapy. *J Clin Gastroenterol.* 1997;25(Suppl 1):S229-34.

30. **Greenlaw R, Sheahan DG, Deluca V, et al.** Gastroduodenitis: a broader concept of peptic ulcer disease. *Dig Dis Sci.* 1980;25:660–72.

31. **McColl KEL, Murray LS, El-Omar E, et al.** Symptomatic benefit from eradicating *Helicobacter pylori* infection in patients with nonulcer dyspepsia. *N Engl J Med.* 1998;26:1869–74.

32. **Blum A, Talley NJ, O'Morain C, et al.** Lack of effect of treating *Helicobacter pylori* infection in patients with nonulcer dyspepsia. *N Engl J Med.* 1998;26:1875–81.

33. **Gisbert JP, Boixeda D, Martin de Argila C, et al.** Erosive duodenitis: prevalence of *Helicobacter pylori* and response to eradication therapy with omeprazole plus two antibiotics. *Eur J Gastroenterol Hepatol.* 1997;9:957–62.

34. **Pace F, Santalucia F, Bianchi Porro G.** Natural history of gastro-oesophageal reflux disease without esophagitis. *Gut.* 1991;32:845–8.

35. **McDougall NI, Johnston BT, Collins A, et al.** Three- to four-and-a-half-year prospective study of prognostic indicators in gastro-oesophageal reflux disease. *Scand J Gastroenterol.* 1998;33:1016–22.

36. **Locke GR, Talley NJ, Fett SL, et al.** Prevalence and clinical spectrum of gastro-esophageal reflux: a population-based study in Olmsted County, Minnesota. *Gastroenterology.* 1997;112:1448–56.

37. **Savary M, Miller G.** *The Oesophagus.* Soluthurn, Switzerland: Gassman; 1977.

38. **Bytzer P, Havelund T, Moller Hansen J.** Interobserver variation in the endoscopic diagnosis of reflux esophagitis. *Scand J Gastroenterol.* 1993;28:119–25.

39. **Lundell L, Dent J, Bennett JR, et al.** Endoscopic assessment of esophagitis: clinical and functional correlates and further validation of the Los Angeles classification. *Gut.* 1999;2:172–80.

40. **Small PK, Loudon MA, Waldron B, et al.** Importance of reflux symptoms in functional dyspepsia. *Gut.* 1995;36:189–92.

41. **Wiener GJ, Richter JE, Copper JB, et al.** The symptom index: a clinically important parameter of ambulatory 24-hour esophageal pH monitoring. *Am J Gastroenterol.* 1988;83:358–61.

42. **Lind T, Havelund T, Carlsson R, et al.** Gastroesophageal reflux disease without esophagitis: efficacy of omeprazole therapy and features determining therapeutic response. *Scand J Gastroenterol.* In press.

43. **Schenk BE, Kuipers EJ, Klinkenberg-Knol EC, et al.** Omeprazole as a diagnostic tool in gastroesophageal reflux disease. *Am J Gastroenterol.* 1997;92:1997–2000.

44. **El-Serag HB, Sonnenberg A.** Opposing time trends of peptic ulcer and reflux disease. *Gut.* 1998;43:327–33.

45. **Cameron AJ, Zinsmeister AR, Ballard DJ, Carney JA.** Prevalence of columnar-lined (Barrett's) esophagus: comparison of population-based clinical and autopsy findings. *Gastroenterology.* 1990;99:918–22.

46. **Doll R, Avery JF, Buckatzsch MM.** *MRC Special Report: Occupational Factors in the Aetiology of Gastric and Duodenal Ulcers, with an Estimate of Their Incidence in the General Population,* series no 276. London; HMSO; 1951.

47. **Weir RD, Backett EM.** Studies of the epidemiology of peptic ulcer in a rural community: prevalence and natural history of dyspepsia and peptic ulcer. *Gut.* 1968;9:75–83.

48. **Jennings D.** Perforated peptic ulcer: changes in age-incidence and sex distribution in the last 150 years. *Lancet.* 1940;1:395–8,444–7.

49. **Fineberg HV, Pearlman LA.** Surgical treatment of peptic ulcer in the U.S.: trends before and after the introduction of cimetidine. *Lancet.* 1981;1:1305–7.

50. **Susser M.** Period effects, generation effects, and age effects in peptic ulcer mortality. *J Chron Dis.* 1982;35:29–40.

51. **Banatvala N, Mayo K, Megraud F, et al.** The cohort effect and *Helicobacter pylori. J Infect Dis.* 1993;168:219–21.

52. **Megraud F.** Epidemiology of *Helicobacter pylori* infection: Where are we in 1995? *Eur J Gastroenterol Hepatol.* 1995;7:292–5.

53. **Christensen A, Bousfield R, Christiansen J.** Incidence of perforated and bleeding ulcers before and after the introduction of H_2-receptor antagonists. *Ann Surg.* 1988;207:4–6.

54. **Makela J, Laitinen S, Kairaluoma MI.** Complications of peptic ulcer disease before and after the introduction of H_2-receptor antagonists. *Hepatogastroenterology.* 1992;39:144–8.

55. **Negre J.** Perforated ulcer in elderly people. *Lancet.* 1985;2:1118–9.

56. **Hermansson M, Stael von Holstein C, Zilling T.** Peptic ulcer perforation before and after the introduction of H_2-receptor blockers and proton pump inhibitors. *Scand J Gastroenterol.* 1997;32:523–9.

57. **Paimela H, Tuompo PK, Perakyl T, et al.** Peptic ulcer surgery in Helsinki from 1972–1987. *Br J Surg.* 1991;78:28–31.

58. **Gustavsson S, Kelly KA, Melton LJ, Zinsmeister AR.** Trends in peptic ulcer surgery. *Gastroenterology.* 1988;94:688–94.

59. **Goodwin CS, Worsley BW.** The *Helicobacter* genus: the history of *H. pylori* and taxonomy of current species. In Goodwin CS, Worsley BW (eds). Helicobacter pylori: *Biology and Clinical Practice.* Boca Raton, FL: CRC Press; 1993:2–13.

60. **Warren JR, Marshall BM.** Unidentified curved bacilli on gastric epithelium in active chronic gastritis. *Lancet.* 1983;1:1273–5.

61. **Megraud F, Brassens-Rabbe MP, Denis F, et al.** Seroepidemiology of *Campylobacter pylori* infection in various populations. *J Clin Microbiol.* 1989;27:1870–3.

62. **Anonymous.** Epidemiology of, and risk factors for, *Helicobacter pylori* infection among 3194 asymptomatic subjects in 17 populations: the Eurogast Study Group. *Gut.* 1993;34:1672–6.

63. **Cave DR.** Transmission and epidemiology of *Helicobacter pylori. Am J Med.* 1996;100:12-8S

64. **Jyotheeswaran S, Shah AN, Jin HO, et al.** Prevalence of *Helicobacter pylori* in peptic ulcer patients in greater Rochester, New York: Is empirical triple therapy justified? *Am J Gastroenterol.* 1998;93:574–8.

65. **Sprung DJ, Apter M, Allen B, et al.** The prevalence of *Helicobacter pylori* in duodenal ulcer disease: a community-based study. *Am J Gastroenterol.* 1996;91:1926.

66. **Henry A, Batey RG.** Low prevalence of *Helicobacter pylori* in an Australian duodenal ulcer population: NSAIDitis or the effect of ten years of *H. pylori* treatment? *Aust N Z J Med.* 1998;28:345.

67. **Nebel OT, Fornes MF, Castell DO.** Symptomatic gastroesophageal reflux: incidence and precipitating factors. *Dig Dis Sci.* 1976;21:953–6.

68. **Ott DJ, McManus CM, Ledbetter MS, et al.** Heartburn correlated to 24-hour pH monitoring and radiographic examination of the esophagus. *Am J Gastroenterol.* 1997;92:1827–30.

69. **Brunnen PL, Karmody AM, Needham CD.** Severe peptic esophagitis. *Gut.* 1969;10:831–7.

70. **Elfberg B.** The incidence of reflux esophagitis. *Scand J Gastroenterol.* 1993;28:113–8.

71. **Blot WJ, Devesa S, Kneller RW, Fraumeni JF.** Rising incidence of adenocarcinoma of the esophagus and gastric cardia. *JAMA.* 1991;265:1287–9.

72. **Labenz J, Blum AL, Bayerdorffer E, et al.** Curing *Helicobacter pylori* infection in patients with duodenal ulcer may provoke reflux esophagitis. *Gastroenterology.* 1997;112:1442–7.

73. **Malferheiner P, Veldhuzen van Zantan S, Dent J, et al.** Does cure of *Helicobacter pylori* infection induce heartburn? (Abstract). *Gastroenterology.* 1998;114:A212.

74. **Talley NJ, Janssens J, Louritsen K, et al.** No increase of reflux symptoms or esophagitis in patients with nonulcer dyspepsia 12 months after *Helicobacter pylori* eradication: a randomized, double-blind, placebo-controlled trial (Abstract). *Gastroenterology.* 1998;114:A306.

75. **Mitchell HM, Hazell SL, Li YY et al.** Serological response to specific *Helicobacter pylori* antigens: antibody against CagA antigen is not predictive of gastric cancer in a developing country. *Am J Gastroenterol.* 1996;91:1785–8.

76. **Kang JY, Tay HH, Yap I, et al.** Low frequency of endoscopic esophagitis in Asian patients. *J Clin Gastroenterol.* 1993;16:70–3.

77. **Ho KY, Ng WL, Kang JY, Yeoh KG.** Gastroesophageal reflux is a common cause of noncardiac chest pain in a country with a low prevalence of reflux esophagitis. *Dig Dis Sci.* 1998;43:1991–7.

78. **Kang JY, Yap I, Gwee KA.** The pattern of functional and organic disorders in an Asian gastroenterological clinic. *J Gastroenterol Hepatol.* 1994;9:124–7.

79. **Ho KY, Kang JY, Viegas OA.** Symptomatic gastroesophageal reflux in pregnancy: a prospective study among Singaporean women. *J Gastroenterol Hep.* 1998;13:1020–6.

80. **Nyren O, Adami HO, Gustavsson S, et al.** The "epigastric distress syndrome": a possible disease entity identified by history and endoscopy in patients with nonulcer dyspepsia. *J Clin Gastroenterol.* 1987;9:303–9.

81. **Richter JE, Falk GW, Vaezi MF.** *Helicobacter pylori* and gastroesophageal reflux disease: the bug may not be all bad. *Am J Gastroenterol.* 1998;93:1800–2.

82. **Sampliner RE.** Adenocarcinoma of the esophagus and gastric cardia: Is there progress in the face of increasing cancer incidence? *Ann Intern Med.* 1999;130:67–9.

83. **Talley NJ, Lam SK, Goh KL, Fock KM.** Management guidelines for uninvestigated and functional dyspepsia in the Asia-Pacific region: First Asian Pacific Working Party on Functional Dyspepsia. *J Gastroenterol Hepatol.* 1998;13:335–53.

84. **Shaw MJ, Kane RL, Fendrick AM, et al.** The impact of over-the-counter histamine-2 antagonists: great expectations unfulfilled (Abstract). *Gastroenterology.* 1998;114:A41.

85. **Shaw MJ, Beebe TJ, et al.** Health care seeking for dyspepsia in a community sample: role of the pain experience, comorbid illness and health-related quality of life (Abstract). *Gastroenterology.* 1998;114;A40.

86. **Forbes GM, Glaser ME, Cullen DJE, et al.** Duodenal ulcer treated with *Helicobacter pylori* eradication: seven-year follow-up. *Lancet.* 1994;343:258–60.

87. **Jorde R, Bostad L, Burhol PG.** Asymptomatic gastric ulcer: a follow-up study in patients with previous gastric ulcer disease. *Lancet.* 1986;1:119–20.

88. **Gilvarry J, Buckley MJ, Beattie S, et al.** Eradication of *Helicobacter pylori* affects symptoms in nonulcer dyspepsia. *Scand J Gastroenterol.* 1997;32:535–40.

89. **Bytzer P, Moller-Hansen J, de Muckadell OBS.** Empirical H_2-blocker therapy or prompt endoscopy in management of dyspepsia. *Lancet.* 1994;343:811–6.

90. **Hansen JM, Bytzer P, Bondesen S, de Muckadell OBS.** Efficacy and outcome of an open access endoscopy service. *Dan Med Bull.* 1991;38:288–90.

91. **Jones R.** What happens to patients with nonulcer dyspepsia after endoscopy? *Practitioner.* 1988;232:75–8.

92. **Ofman JJ, Rabeneck L.** The effectiveness of endoscopy in the management of dyspepsia: a qualitative systematic review. *Am J Med.* 1999;106:335–46.

93. **Blustein PK, Beck PL, Meddings JB, et al.** The utility of endoscopy in the management of patients with gastroesophageal reflux symptoms. *Am J Gastroenterol.* 1998;93:2508–12.

94. **Talley NJ.** Dyspepsia. *Ballieres Clin Gastroenterol.* 1998;12:3,418,624.

95. **McColl KEL, El-Nujumi A, El-Omar E, et al.** The *Helicobacter pylori* breath test: a surrogate marker for peptic ulcer disease in dyspeptic patients. *Gut.* 1997;40:302–6.

96. **Patel P, Khulusi S, Mendall MA, et al.** Prospective screening of dyspeptic patients by *Helicobacter pylori* serology. *Lancet.* 1995;346:1315–8.

97. **Duggan A, Elliott C, Logan RPH, et al.** Does 'near-patient' *H. pylori* testing in primary care reduce referral for endoscopy?: results from a randomised trial (Abstract). *Gastroenterology.* 1998;114:A110.

2

Initial Management of Unexplained Dyspepsia Without Alarm Symptoms: Empirical Therapy or Endoscopy?

M. Brian Fennerty, MD

Dyspepsia occurs frequently in an otherwise healthy population. As many as 25% to 40% of adult individuals will experience symptoms of dyspepsia in a given year (5–10); however, most dyspepsia patients do not seek medical attention for these symptoms. The reasons why individuals with dyspepsia seeks health care for this symptom complex is unclear, but it is likely due in part to an underlying concern about having a serious disease (11,12). Even though only a minority of patients with dyspepsia seeks medical attention, 4% to 5% of all primary care physician office visits are for dyspepsia complaints (5). Therefore, dyspepsia and its management are important clinical issues to both primary care physicians and gastroenterologists (13).

Dyspepsia can indicate the presence of a variety of pathologic processes, such as duodenal ulcer, gastric ulcer, nonulcer dyspepsia (NUD), cholelithiasis, gastroesophageal reflux disease (GERD), gastroparesis, other upper gut motility abnormalities, "visceral hyperalgesia," and gastric cancer. An attempt has been made to categorize symptoms of dyspepsia into subgroups ("ulcer-like," "reflux-like," "dysmotility-like," and "other") to improve the diagnostic accuracy of the associated symptoms (14). Unfortunately, subsequent studies using this classification system have indicated that the use of subgroups was not predictive of the underlying disease process (15). Moreover, many patients exhibit more than one symptom subgroup and overlap with irritable bowel symptoms (16). Thus, a definitive diagnosis of the underlying disease process cannot be made based on the history alone in a patient presenting to his or her physician with symptoms of dyspepsia but without alarm symptoms (e.g., weight loss, vomiting, bleeding) or symptoms or signs of gastric outlet obstruction (15). The clinician must carefully review the history for drugs that can cause dyspeptic symptoms, such as nonsteroidal anti-inflammatory drugs (NSAIDs), aspirin, and antibiotics. A careful review of the side-effect profiles of all drugs is paramount, because many can cause gastrointestinal symptoms. If systemic disease (e.g., diabetes, scleroderma, renal failure, intestinal obstruction) has been ruled out, alarm symptoms are not present, and the physical examination is normal (as it almost always is, because the examination is not usually helpful unless an abdominal mass is present), then the clinician is faced with a direct choice: Should the patient be treated empirically or be evaluated endoscopically to rule out organic diseases? (An upper GI series is not an effective option because the sensitivity and specificity are unacceptably low compared with endoscopy.)

In an era in which efficiency in the management of health care resources is emphasized, the optimal diagnostic approach to dyspepsia is not clear. This chapter explores various initial diagnostic and management approaches and attempts to determine whether endoscopic management or a "trial of therapy" is the most appropriate initial treatment strategy in a patient presenting with symptoms of dyspepsia.

Diagnostic Findings

In patients with dyspepsia who are referred for endoscopy, approximately 15% to 20% are found to have peptic ulcer disease (PUD), 15% to 20% esophagitis, 5% to 40% gastritis or duodenitis, and 1% gastric cancer (5). The rest of these individuals are classified as having nonulcer dyspepsia (NUD), although 15% to 20% probably have endoscopy-negative reflux disease (ENRD). This prevalence of ENRD is based on the extrapolation of data that indicates that only 40% to 50% of patients with GERD have erosive esophagitis; thus, GERD may be a more prevalent causative factor of dyspepsia (30%–40%) than PUD (15%–20%). Nevertheless, 50% or more of patients with dyspepsia fall into the category of NUD. Therefore, although the association between PUD, GERD, gastric cancer, and dyspeptic symptoms seems intuitively obvious, the mechanisms that produce dyspepsia are less clear in the 50% or more of patients that have NUD. Numerous potential mechanisms for symptoms in patients with NUD have been postulated, and some or all of them may be valid (3,17,18,19). Some patients seem to have an acid-sensitive mucosa despite the absence of ulcers or GERD; others may demonstrate disordered gastroduodenal motility or visceral hyperalgesia or may have symptoms related to mucosal inflammation or a combination of these factors. For example, in a *Helicobacter pylori*-infected individual, dyspepsia could result from 1) an *H. pylori*-induced ulcer, 2) an effect of the associated inflammatory reaction without concomitant ulceration, 3) secondary to inflammation-induced disordered gastric motility, 4) a change in receptor activity, or 5) a combination of these or other unknown factors. Similarly, most patients with ulcer-like dyspepsia do not have an ulcer; moreover, some of these patients do not respond to the usual antisecretory therapy used to treat ulcer-induced dyspepsia. Thus, a precise endoscopic diagnosis of PUD, NUD, *H. pylori* gastritis, etc. may not necessarily indicate the optimal therapeutic approach. Furthermore, therapeutic trials aimed at decreasing acid production or eradicating *H. pylori* infection are not effective in relieving symptoms in all dyspepsia patients; hence, a single management approach is unlikely to be appropriate for all dyspepsia patients (Fig. 2.1).

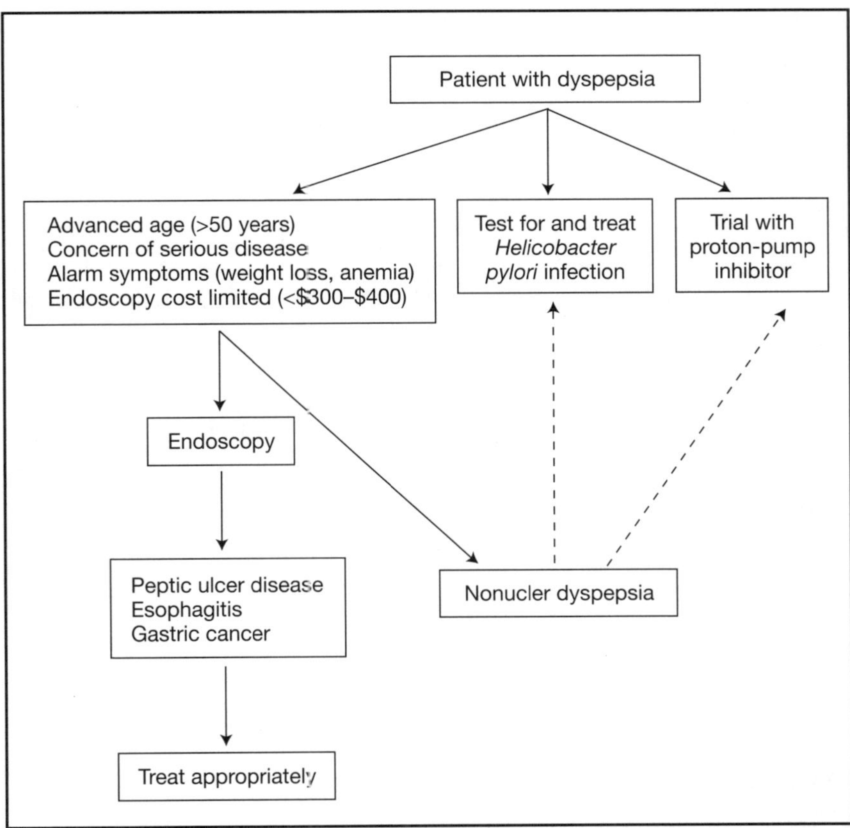

Figure 2.1   One possible initial management strategy for a patient with dyspepsia.

Endoscopy in the Initial Management of Dyspepsia

What is the role of endoscopy in patients presenting with dyspepsia? If endoscopy was inexpensive, nonmorbid, office based, and universally available, it would always be used initially to investigate a patient presenting with dyspepsia because it is the most accurate means of diagnosing duodenal ulcer, gastric ulcer, gastric cancer, esophagitis, and NUD (5). Prompt use of endoscopy to investigate dyspepsia would then lead to a recommendation of specific therapy for certain indications (i.e., ulcers, esophagitis, cancer, and *H. pylori* infection) or would signify that symptomatic trials should be attempted for other indications (i.e., NUD). However, despite the effect of RBRVS (resource-based relative value scale) reimbursement and the emergence of managed care cost containment, the cost and invasiveness of endoscopy continue to limit its use as an initial management strategy for dyspepsia. Is this limitation justified?

Advantages and Disadvantages

What are the advantages and disadvantages of using endoscopy in a patient presenting with dyspepsia? (Table 2.1). Endoscopy is the most accurate means of diagnosing most diseases of the gastrointestinal mucosa, including those associated with symptoms of dyspepsia (e.g., ulcer disease, esophagitis, gastric cancer). In these cases, a definitive diagnosis is obtained and a clear, evidence-based treatment plan can be formulated. The presence of ulcers caused by *H. pylori* or the use of NSAIDs can be ascertained and treated appropriately. In *H. pylori*-negative, NSAID-negative ul-

Table 2.1   Endoscopy in the Initial Management of Dyspepsia

Advantages

- Definitive diagnosis

- Reassurance value

- Possible increased patient satisfaction

Disadvantages

- Cost

- Invasiveness

- Generally not office based

- Possible referral requirement

cer cases, antisecretory agents (e.g., H_2-receptor antagonists [H2RAs] or proton-pump inhibitors [PPIs]) have proved effective in healing, symptom relief, and maintenance of remission in most patients. In patients with gastric cancer, staging can be determined and appropriate therapy can be prescribed. One disadvantage is that most patients with dyspepsia will have either a normal endoscopic examination (i.e., NUD) or lesions that may not be directly responsible for dyspepsia (e.g., inflammation, erythema, or erosions). However, one could argue that the diagnosis of NUD is, in fact, specific and therefore an appropriate therapeutic plan of symptomatic treatment can be outlined in these patients as well.

Patient Reassurance

Reassurance and patient satisfaction are other potential advantages of endoscopy, but unfortunately these patient-centered outcomes have not been well studied (20–23). However, data indicate that reassurance of the lack of serious disease and/or improved patient satisfaction may in fact occur in patients with dyspepsia who undergo endoscopy (24,25). Although empirical therapy is a time-honored practice in primary care and the standard of care for many symptomatic complaints (e.g., dysuria, pharyngitis, low back pain), it is likely that some dyspepsia patients may not be satisfied with a strategy that is akin to the clinician saying, "I'm pretty sure I know what it is, so I am going to treat you with this." In other words, patients with either an expressed or underlying fear of serious disease (e.g., cancer, PUD) may wish for a definitive diagnosis and may be dissatisfied unless one is obtained (11). Surprisingly, no studies have investigated this concept specifically, yet there is indirect evidence that some patients do express dissatisfaction with vague diagnoses.

Bytzer and coworkers (24) evaluated the presence or absence of symptoms, use of health care resources, costs, sick leave, and satisfaction in dyspepsia patients who were treated either empirically or referred immediately for endoscopy. In this population-based study, 77 out of 106 general practitioners in Odense, Denmark, referred 414 patients with dyspepsia into this study. Two hundred eight of these patients were randomized to receive a prompt endoscopy, and the other 206 received empirical H2RA therapy (ranitidine 150 mg bid) plus endoscopy if therapy failed or symptoms recurred. Of those receiving prompt endoscopy, 37% had organic disease (which is similar to previous study findings). There was an identical yield of organic disease in those in the empirical-therapy arm who later received endoscopy (66% of these underwent the later endoscopy because of relapse or symptomatic recurrence). At 1 year, there were no differences in dyspeptic symptoms or quality of life between the two treatment groups. However, the group receiving initial empirical therapy demonstrated increased costs secondary to an increase in sick days taken, physician visits, and drug costs.

In the group that was initially treated empirically but that later underwent endoscopy, there was a 20-fold increase in the use of sick days, indicating that a delayed definitive diagnosis in this subgroup resulted in greatly increased expenditures for the entire empirically treated group. Although, it was not specifically investigated in this study, perhaps these patients were the ones who had a perception that their symptoms indicated something serious. Additionally, the patients randomized to receive initial endoscopy management exhibited greater satisfaction in their care, with 94% being satisfied or very satisfied with their care compared with only 53% in those in the empirical-therapy group. Thus, although symptom outcome remained equivalent, patient satisfaction improved, which perhaps was related to a decreased concern about a "missed or serious disease."

This hypothesis about the reassurance value of endoscopy is also supported, in part, by the fact that up to 40% of dyspepsia patients seeking an evaluation from their general practitioner express fear of a serious or potentially fatal disease (11). Thus, a normal endoscopy may have reassurance value, may increase overall sense of well being, and may even improve outcome. Psychosocial factors may influence who presents for health care and who benefits most from an endoscopic examination. This is an area in which further study is warranted.

A recent study by Wiklund and coworkers (25) indirectly supports the reassurance value of endoscopy. As part of a placebo-controlled, double-blind, randomized trial comparing omeprazole versus placebo in consecutive dyspeptic patients referred to a gastrointestinal specialist, the effect of endoscopy on quality of life was ascertained. One hundred ninety-six patients who had not yet received treatment for dyspepsia were investigated with three validated quality-of-life instruments (the Psychologic General Well-Being Score (PGWB), Gastrointestinal Symptoms Rating Scale (GSRS), and SF-36 Quality-of-Life Instrument) before and 1 week after endoscopy. Baseline quality-of-life data in these patients were worse than in normal individuals, and symptoms remained unchanged after their endoscopic examinations. However, quality of life normalized 1 week after endoscopy in many patients even though all had negative endoscopic findings and remained symptomatic. These data suggest that patients who consult physicians for dyspepsia are self-selected and differ from nonconsulting community patients. One could speculate that perhaps, in this subgroup, negative endoscopic examinations may lead to not only an improved quality of life but to decreased subsequent health care use as well.

Further supporting the reassurance value of endoscopy—and the role of specialty consultation in the initial management approach—are data from Longstreth (26). In this study, 6-month costs of managing dyspepsia were evaluated in those receiving a gastrointestinal consult and endoscopy versus those receiving a barium study and primary care evaluation. The cost for patients referred for consultation and endoscopy was $134 compared with $435 for those treated in a primary care setting.

All of the above data, which favor the hypothesis that endoscopy provides reassurance, are contradicted by only one study (26a) (*see also* Chapter 8, reference 38). Unfortunately, improvement in quality of life or patient satisfaction has never been tested in an appropriately designed clinical trial. Given recent data about *H. pylori* treatment and PPI therapy in patients with NUD, an appropriately designed trial that uses validated symptom and quality-of-life instruments with adequate follow-up and that randomly selects patients for endoscopy versus a trial of PPI and/or *H. pylori* therapy is necessary to discover whether endoscopy is an appropriate initial management strategy in patients with dyspepsia. Despite the lack of an appropriately designed study, initial evaluation by endoscopy still may be a relevant option (*see* Fig. 2.1).

Are Previously Published Guidelines About Endoscopy Still Relevant?

Current American College of Physicians (ACP) guidelines (established in 1985, but now undergoing revision and no longer considered official policy) relegate endoscopy to a secondary position in dyspepsia patients (27). Other associations (e.g., the European Working Party on Dyspepsia) came up with similar recommendations in 1988 (28). The rationale for ACP's recommendation was that potentially fatal disease (gastric cancer) was found in only 1% of patients presenting with dyspepsia, and of these patients only 10% (0.1% of all patients with dyspepsia) had early-stage gastric cancer in which a cure is possible. Thus, early endoscopy in an effort to prevent cancer deaths made little sense if this was the primary reason for its use, especially given its associated cost. Instead, a trial of therapy with an H2RA for 6 to 8 weeks was recommended, with endoscopy reserved for those with no response after 7 to 10 days or those with recurrent symptoms following the conclusion of therapy. It is important to consider that at the time these guidelines were created, the standard of care in treating PUD (and other common upper gastrointestinal conditions) was 6 to 8 weeks of an H2RA. Therefore, because cancer was rarely curable and PUD would be treated adequately with this recommended empirical approach, this initial management strategy made intuitive sense. However, patients that were not expected to respond to a trial of an H2RA (e.g., those with NUD or with lesions that should respond) and those that were expected to develop recurrent symptoms at the conclusion of therapy (e.g., those with PUD or GERD) would still be examined with endoscopy. Thus, these guidelines merely postponed the inevitable because many, if not most, dyspepsia patients would eventually receive an endoscopic examination anyway!

Since that time, the role of *H. pylori* and NSAIDs in causing most cases of PUD has been clarified. Thus, an accurate endoscopic diagnosis of an *H.*

pylori- or NSAID-associated ulcer may dictate a specific therapy that offers a chance to "cure" PUD by curing the underlying *H. pylori* infection or by discontinuing NSAID use. Similarly, some patients with GERD require PPI therapy for symptom relief and remission maintenance. However, because PPIs were not available when these guidelines were developed, this therapeutic "need" was not appreciated. Thus, not only are the 1985 guidelines counterproductive to their intent of decreasing the use of endoscopy, they do not take into account therapies other than H_2 receptor–antagonist trial for complicated GERD, *H. pylori*-related diseases (PUD, NUD[?]), and the NSAID-related gastroduodenal disease that has emerged since that time. Whether endoscopy's role also has changed since those recommendations were published remains to be determined.

Empirical Trials in the Initial Management of Dyspepsia

Is there a role for a trial of therapy in the initial management of dyspepsia? Most of the interest in this initial management approach has concerned the trials of *H. pylori* therapy in infected patients with NUD (29–35). This interest is related to a modest increase in the prevalence of *H. pylori* in dyspepsia patients (19). However, a causative relationship between *H. pylori* dyspepsia is not yet established. Furthermore, there are few data from controlled clinical trials on which to decide whether therapy is effective for symptom relief. However, some dyspeptic patients infected with *H. pylori* undoubtedly have PUD. A trial of empirical therapy benefiting even these few dyspeptic patients with *H. pylori* ulcers could lead to overall benefits for the entire group, even if symptom relief is not achieved in the other NUD patients.

Decision Analysis

Because of the lack of controlled trial data, the role of an *H. pylori* "test and treat" strategy in dyspepsia has been studied by means of decision analysis (36–41). Clinical decision analysis is a quantitative technique used systematically to evaluate management strategies when data from randomized controlled trials are not available on which to base clinical recommendations. Instead, available data from the literature and expert opinion are used to establish probabilities of specific treatment outcomes, and costs can be derived through a roll-back technique. Unfortunately, because all decision-analysis models use some assumptions in their construction, different models investigating the same clinical issue may yield dissimilar results.

Fendrick and coworkers (36) were the first to use decision analysis to ascertain the most appropriate initial management strategy for the dyspepsia patient with suspected PUD. Five management strategies were analyzed: 1) *H. pylori* "test and treat" strategy, 2) immediate endoscopy with biopsy, 3) immediate endoscopy without biopsy, 4) empirical treatment with *H. pylori* therapy, and 5) empirical treatment with an H2RA. In this model, all three nonendoscopic strategies were more cost effective in the base-case scenario. Using sensitivity analysis, it was determined that the cost of endoscopy and the rate of recurrent dyspepsia symptoms were the key variables that affected outcome. In the base case, it was assumed that the cost of endoscopy was $1180 and that the recurrence of dyspepsia symptoms would occur in 30% of patients. When costs of endoscopy fell and/or the recurrence of dyspepsia symptoms was more frequent, then an initial endoscopic management strategy became the most cost-effective one. Although this analysis did not identify the optimal strategy for managing dyspepsia, it did emphasize that the cost of an endoscopy was paramount in determining what should be the preferred management option. In this analysis, when the cost of endoscopy fell below $500, it achieved a cost effectiveness that was equivalent with nonendoscopic strategies. Interestingly, this cost is not much different than the cost of endoscopy in many regions of the United States today. However, these data also indicate that where endoscopy remains expensive, an *H. pylori* "test and treat" strategy is the most cost effective.

Silverstein and coworkers (37) used decision analysis to investigate the optimal initial management strategy in a patient with new-onset dyspepsia. They concluded that there was only a 1.8% difference in the cost between an initial endoscopic strategy compared with empirical therapy in this situation. The difference between these models' conclusions is explained in part by the use of different assumptions that highlight the "pitfalls" of decision analysis.

Ofman and coworkers (38) used decision analysis to conclude that the cost of endoscopy would need to decrease 90% or more for it to be as cost effective as a "test and treat" strategy (38). Rubin and coworkers (39) used decision analysis to determine that a "test and treat" strategy for patients with dyspepsia was less costly (by 17%) than endoscopy but that it resulted in more symptomatic days.

Numerous other decision-analysis models also have been published. Sonnenberg (40) concluded that an initial "test and treat" strategy is cost effective in patients with dyspepsia so long as 10% or more of the dyspepsia patients have *H. pylori* ulcers. This model assumed there was no benefit for NUD patients infected with *H. pylori* who were treated. Despite this, there was an overall clinical benefit because of the enormous benefit obtained in the few patients with *H. pylori* ulcers. However, it is estimated that it may take as long as 5 to 18 years for this strategy to attain its cost benefit, and Read and coworkers (41) supported an individual approach based on this estimate. These studies also ignored the potential harm in eradicating *H. pylori*. Because *H. pylori* infection may result in either a decrease (or buffering) of gastric acid, perhaps eradication may increase the incidence of other acid-related disease or may inhibit the efficacy of PPI antisecretory therapy. Although data are inconclusive, *H. pylori* infection may decrease the incidence of GERD, NSAID gastropathy, or both (42–45).

Determining the optimal strategy of managing dyspepsia patients will remain controversial until we have performed properly designed studies that investigate endoscopy versus an *H. pylori* "test and treat" strategy, with an evaluation of appropriate clinical and economic outcomes. In the meantime, however, these studies do indicate that endoscopy becomes a more reasonable initial strategy option as its costs decrease.

Empirical *Helicobacter pylori* Therapy

As discussed in the preceding section, decision analysis was used because of the lack of controlled-trial data about dyspepsia-patient management. However, there have been some recent clinical trials on the effects of testing for and treating *H. pylori* in patients with NUD. It is important, however, that the data from these trials be viewed in an appropriate context. All of the patients in these trials had undergone an endoscopic evaluation before treatment. Thus, outcomes of these studies cannot be used to determine the optimal initial approach. However, these data do add to our overall knowledge about possible outcomes of different management strategies.

Two studies on treating *H. pylori* infection in patients with NUD—one by Blum and coworkers (46), the other by McColl and coworkers (47)—differ in their conclusions. In each of these trials, well-characterized patients with NUD were randomized to receive either *H. pylori* therapy or PPI antisecretory therapy alone. Using validated dyspepsia instruments, follow-up over 1 year showed a significant difference in outcome between those treated for *H. pylori* compared with the control group in McColl's study, whereas the Blum study showed no difference in outcome. However, perhaps most important was that only approximately 25% of patients treated for *H. pylori* in either study were symptom-free at the end of 1 year, and even fewer were symptom-free after a single course of PPI therapy. Thus, even if an *H. pylori* "test and treat" strategy is clinically more effective, the benefit of this strategy is likely modest at best in patients with NUD. Because NUD is the diagnosis in most dyspepsia patients, one may question the efficacy of empirical *H. pylori* trials in this situation.

Empirical Antisecretory Therapy

What about the role of empirical antisecretory therapy? Although H2RAs are effective in the symptom relief and healing of approximately 80% of patients with PUD, they are much less effective in healing or relieving symptoms of GERD. Because 15% to 20% of dyspepsia patients have objective evidence of GERD (i.e., esophagitis) and given that less than half of the patients with GERD have esophagitis, it can be assumed that as many as 30% to 40% of dyspepsia patients may have GERD and another 10% to 20% may have PUD. Given the quicker and superior symptom relief with a PPI compared with an H2RA in these two groups of patients, it makes intuitive sense that a PPI may be more effective in a therapeutic trial than an H2RA in dyspepsia patients (48). Unfortunately, there are few data about the effectiveness of antisecretory therapy in dyspepsia patients (49). The study in which Bytzer and coworkers (24) compared prompt endoscopy with a trial of an H2RA has been discussed already. More recently, Laheij and coworkers (50) compared the outcome at 1 year in dyspepsia patients randomized to receive prompt endoscopy or a 2- to 4-week trial of omeprazole with reinstitution of omeprazole for 8 weeks for relapses. Only 31% of patients treated empirically with omeprazole later underwent endoscopy, and overall costs were less in the empirical group than in the endoscopic group ($284 and $491, respectively). These data indicate that perhaps empirical antisecretory therapy may be an effective initial-management option if a more potent antisecretory agent is used. Recently, Talley and coworkers (51) also evaluated this management approach in patients with NUD. In their study, an empirical trial of PPI therapy also was found to be more effective in patients with NUD. However, as with the above therapeutic trials performed in *H. pylori*-infected NUD patients discussed in the previous section, the overall effect on symptoms was modest.

Conclusions

How are dyspepsia patients initially managed most effectively? Better yet, who should undergo definitive diagnostic testing and who should have an empirical trial of therapy? Not surprisingly, there is no one best answer using evidence-based analysis of the literature. Instead, a variety of initial management options can be justified at this time, and the management of dyspepsia remains part of the "art" of practicing medicine. However, as discussed below in the "Recommendations" section, there are circumstances in which a specific approach may be preferable. Thus, either an empirical trial of therapy or an initial diagnostic evaluation with endoscopy can be a prudent initial management strategy depending on the clinical situation. In the future, one strategy may become dominant if properly conducted trials are performed, but in the meantime physician and patient preference should determine the initial management strategy for dyspepsia.

Recommendations

- In the stable, healthy patient, under 50 to 55 years of age who expresses no concern of underlying serious disease, an office-based antibody test for *H. pylori* infection (and subsequent treatment for those who test positive) should be considered. In those testing negative for *H. pylori* infection, a 4- to 8-week trial of therapy with a PPI may be useful.

- Prompt endoscopy is recommended for older individuals with dyspepsia, those who express a concern about serious disease, and patients in whom the clinician suspects serious disease.

- In regions or situations in which endoscopy costs have been decreased markedly, prompt endoscopy may be appealing for a broad range of patients.

Key Points

- Approximately half of all patients who undergo endoscopy for dyspepsia are found to have no organic cause of their symptoms. These patients are categorized as having nonulcer dyspepsia.

- Although endoscopy is the most accurate means of diagnosing the organic diseases that underlie dyspepsia, the cost and invasiveness of this test limit its use as an initial management strategy.

- The advantages of prompt endoscopy include obtaining a definitive diagnosis that enables the clinician to form a clear and appropriate treatment plan and results in patient reassurance. However, one disadvantage is that endoscopy yields normal results in at least half of all patients.

- Based on the results of several decision analyses, the *H. pylori* "test and treat" strategy is considered more cost effective than endoscopy. These same studies also suggest that in regions where endoscopy costs are low, it should be the preferred management strategy. Nevertheless, more properly designed studies comparing endoscopy and empirical therapy are needed.

REFERENCES

1. **Barbara L, Camilleri M, Corinaldesi GP, et al.** Definition and investigation of dyspepsia: consensus of an international ad hoc working party. *Dig Dis Sci.* 1989; 34:1272–6.

2. **Drossman DA, Thompson WG, Talley NJ, et al.** Identification of subgroups of functional gastrointestinal disorders. *Gastroenterol Int.* 1990;3:159–72.

3. **Talley NJ, Phillips SF.** Nonulcer dyspepsia: potential causes and pathophysiology, *Ann Intern Med.* 1988;108:865–79.

4. AGA technical review: evaluation of dyspepsia. *Gastroenterology.* 1998;114:582–95.

5. **American Gastroenterological Association.** Medical position statement: evaluation of dyspepsia. *Gastroenterology.* 1998;114:579–81.

6. **Knill-Jones RP.** Geographical differences in the prevalence of dyspepsia. *Scand J Gastroenterol.* 1991;26(Suppl 182):17–24.

7. **Talley NJ, Weaver AL, Zinsmeister AR, et al.** Onset and disappearance of gastrointestinal symptoms and functional gastrointestinal disorders. *Am J Epidemiol.* 1992;15:165–77.

8. **Drossman DA, Li Z, Andruzzi E, et al.** U.S. householder survey of functional gastrointestinal disorders: prevalence, sociodemography, and health impact. *Dig Dis Sci.* 1993;38:1569–80.

9. **Jones RH, Lydeard SE, Hobbs FD, et al.** Dyspepsia in England and Scotland. *Gut.* 1990;31:401–5.

10. **Penston JG, Pounder RE.** A survey of dyspepsia in Great Britain. *Aliment Pharmacol Ther.* 1996;10:83–9.

11. **Lydeard S, Jones R.** Factors affecting the decision to consult with dyspepsia: comparison of consulters and nonconsulters. *J R Coll Gen Pract.* 1989;39:495–8.

12. **Holtmann G, Goebell H, Talley NJ.** Dyspepsia in consulters and nonconsulters: prevalence, healthcare seeking behavior and risk factors. *Eur J Gastroenterol Hepatol.* 1994;6:917–24.

13. **Talley NJ, McNeil D, Hayden A, et al.** Prognosis of chronic unexplained dyspepsia. *Gastroenterology.* 1987;92:1060–6.

14. **Talley NJ, Zinsmeister AR, Schleck CD, Melton LJ.** Dyspepsia and dyspepsia subgroups: a population-based study. *Gastroenterology.* 1992;102:1259–68.

15. **Talley NJ, Weaver AL, Tesmer DL, Zinmeister AR.** Lack of discriminant value of dyspepsia subgroups in patients referred for upper endoscopy. *Gastroenterology.* 1993;105:1378–86.

16. **Agreus L, Svardsudd K, Nyren O, Tibblin G.** Irritable bowel syndrome and dyspepsia in the general population: overlap and lack of stability over time. *Gastroenterology.* 1995;109:671–80.

17. **Malagelada JR, Stanghellini V.** Manometric evaluation of functional upper gut symptoms. *Gastroenterology.* 1985;88:1223–31.

18. **Lemann M, Dedering JP, Flourie B, et al.** Abnormal perception of visceral pain in response to gastric distention in chronic idiopathic dyspepsia: the irritable stomach syndrome. *Dig Dis Sci.* 1991;36:1249–56.

19. **Armstrong D.** *Helicobacter pylori* infection and dyspepsia. *Scand J Gastroenterol.* 1996;215(Suppl):38–47.

20. **Williams B, Luckas M, Ellingham JH, et al.** Do young patients with dyspepsia need investigation? *Lancet.* 1988;2:1349–51.

21. **Bytzer P, Schaffalitzky de Muckadell OB.** Prediction of major pathologic conditions in dyspeptic patients referred for endoscopy: a prospective validation study of a scoring system. *Scand J Gastroenterol.* 1992;27:987–92.

22. **Jones R, Lydeard S.** Dyspepsia in the community: a follow-up study. *Br J Clin. Pract* 1992;46:95–7.

23. **Mann J, Holdstock G, Harman M, et al.** Scoring system to improve cost effectiveness of open access endoscopy. *BMJ.* 1983;287:937–40.

24. **Bytzer P, Hansen JM, Schaffalitzky de Muckadell OB.** Empirical H_2-blocker therapy or prompt endoscopy in management of dyspepsia. *Lancet.* 1994;343:811–6.

25. **Wiklund I, Glise H, Jerndal P, et al.** Does endoscopy have a positive impact on quality of life in dyspepsia? *Gastrointest Endosc.* 1998;47:449–54.

26. **Longstreth GF.** Long-term costs after gastroenterology consultation with endoscopy versus radiography in dyspepsia. *Gastrointest Endosc.* 1992;38:23–6.

26a. **Hirth RA, Bloom BS, Chernew ME, Fendrick AM.** Willingness to pay for diagnostic certainty: a comparison among patients, physicians, and managers. *J Gen Intern Med.* 1999;14:193–5.

27. **Health and Public Policy Committee.** Endoscopy in the evaluation of dyspepsia. *Ann Intern Med.* 1985;102:266–9.

28. **Colin-Jones D, Bloom B, Bodemar G, et al.** Management of dyspepsia: report of a working party. *Lancet.* 1988;1:576–9.

29. **Talley NJ.** A critique of therapeutic trials in *Helicobacter pylori*-positive functional dyspepsia. *Gastroenterology.* 1994;106:1174–83.

30. **Laheij RJF, Jansen JBMJ, van de Lisdonk EH, et al.**. Review article: symptom improvement through eradication of *Helicobacter pylori* in patients with nonulcer dyspepsia. *Aliment Pharmacol Ther.* 1996;10:843–50.

31. **Sheu BS, Lin CY, Lin XZ, et al.** Long-term outcome of triple therapy in *Helicobacter pylori*-related nonulcer dyspepsia: a prospective controlled assessment. *Am J Gastroenterol.* 1996;91:441–7.

32. **Veldhuyzen van Zanten SJO, Sherman PM.** *Helicobacter pylori* infection as a cause of gastritis, duodenal ulcer, gastric cancer and nonulcer dyspepsia: a systematic overview. *CMAJ.* 1994;150:177–85.

33. **Elta GH, Scheiman JM, Barnett JL, et al.** Long-term follow-up of *Helicobacter pylori* treatment in nonulcer dyspepsia patients. *Am J Gastroenterol.* 1995;90:1089–93.

34. **McCarthy CO, Patchett S, Collins RM, et al.** Long-term prospective study of *Helicobacter pylori* in nonulcer dyspepsia. *Dig Dis Sci.* 1995;40:114–9.

35. **Holcombe C, Thom C, Kaluba J, et al.** *Helicobacter pylori* clearance in the treatment of nonulcer dyspepsia. *Aliment Pharmacol Therap.* 1992;6:119–23.

36. **Fendrick AM, Chernew ME, Hirth RA, et al.** Alternative management strategies for patients with suspected peptic ulcer disease. *Ann Intern Med.* 1995;123:260–8.

37. **Silverstein MD, Paterson T, Talley NJ.** Initial endoscopy or empirical therapy with or without testing for *Helicobacter pylori* for dyspepsia: a decision analysis. *Gastroenterology.* 1996;110:72–83.

38. **Ofman JJ, Atchison J, Fullerton S, et al.** Management strategies for *Helicobacter pylori*-seropositive patients with dyspepsia: clinical and economic consequences. *Ann Intern Med.* 1997;126:289–91.

39. **Rubin RJ, Cascade EF, Barker RC, et al.** Management of dyspepsia: a decision-analysis model. *Am J Man Care.* 1996;2:647–55.

40. **Sonnenberg A.** Cost-benefit analysis of testing for *Helicobacter pylori* in dyspeptic subjects. *Am J Gastroenterol.* 1996;91:1773–7.

41. **Read L, Pass TM, Komaroff AL.** Diagnosis and treatment of dyspepsia: a cost-effectiveness analysis. *Med Decis Making.* 1982;2:415–38.

42. **Hawkey CJ, Karrasch JA, Szczepanski L, et al.** Omeprazole compared with misoprostol for ulcers and associated with nonsteroidal anti-inflammatory drugs. *N Engl J Med.* 1998;338:727–34.

43. **Yeomans ND, Tulassay Z, Juhasz L, et al.** A comparison of omeprazole with ranitidine for ulcers associated with nonsteroidal anti-inflammatory drugs. *N Engl J Med.* 1998;338:719–26.

44. **Labenz J, Blum AL, Bayerdorffer E, et al.** Curing *Helicobacter pylori* infection in patients with duodenal ulcer may provoke reflux esophagitis. *Gastroenterology.* 1997;112:1442–7.

45. **Vicari JJ, Peek RM, Falk GW, et al.** The seroprevalence of CagA-positive *Helicobacter pylori* strains in the spectrum of the gastroesophageal reflux disease. *Gastroenterology.*1998;115:50–7.

46. **Blum AL, Talley NJ, O'Morain C et al.** Lack of effect of treating *Helicobacter pylori* infection in patients with nonulcer dyspepsia. N Engl J Med 1998;339:1875–81.

47. **McColl K, Murray L, El-Omar E, et al.** Symptomatic benefit from eradicating *Helicobacter pylori. N Engl J Med.* 1998;339:1869–74.

48. **Jones RH, Baxter G.** Lansoprazole 30 mg daily versus ranitidine 150 mg bid in the treatment of acid-related dyspepsia in general practice. *Aliment Pharmacol Ther.* 1997;11:541–6.

49. **Nyren O, Adami HO, Bates S, et al.** Absence of therapeutic benefit from antacids or cimetidine in nonulcer dyspepsia. *N Engl J Med.* 1986;314:339–43.

50. **Laheij RJF, Severens JL, Van de Lisdonk EH, et al.** Randomized controlled trial of omeprazole or endoscopy in patients with persistent dyspepsia: a cost-effectiveness analysis. *Aliment Pharmacol Ther.* 1998;12:1249–56.

51. **Talley NJ, Meineche-Schmidt V, Pare P, et al.** Efficacy of omeprazole in functional dyspepsia: double-blind, randomized, placebo-controlled trials: the Bond and Opera studies. *Aliment Pharmacol Ther.* 1998:12:1055–65.

3

Gastroesophageal Reflux Disease and Dyspepsia

Philip O. Katz, MD

Heartburn occurs daily in 7% to 10% of the U.S. population, and weekly to monthly in 25% to 50% (1–3). Heartburn is often accompanied by regurgitation—the spontaneous appearance of an acid or bitter taste in the chest or mouth. When these classic symptoms of gastroesophageal reflux disease (GERD) are present in the patient with dyspepsia, reflux is likely to be the etiology. Neither the frequency nor the severity of heartburn correlates with that of GERD. Severe disease, including Barrett's esophagus and peptic strictures, may present with infrequent or absent complaints of heartburn, whereas many patients with daily heartburn will have no endoscopic abnormalities. Many patients with atypical manifestations of GERD, including dyspepsia, cough, asthma, or hoarseness, have minimal to no heartburn; therefore, the absence of heartburn does not rule out GERD.

Pathogenesis

The pathogenesis of GERD is multifactorial. Abnormalities include a defective antireflux barrier, abnormal esophageal clearance, altered esophageal mucosal resistance, and delayed gastric emptying. Esophageal injury is

"

caused principally by gastric acid, pepsin, and possibly duodenogastric (bile) reflux.

Abnormalities of the antireflux barrier include hypotensive resting lower esophageal (LES) pressure, transient LES relaxation (TLESR), and hiatal hernia. Inappropriate TLESR—a drop in LES pressure below gastric pressure not accompanied by a swallow—is the most common cause of reflux episodes, reportedly being responsible 65% to 90% of the time (4). Although the mechanism of TLESRs is not clear, one major stimulus is gastric distention; thus, the avoidance of eating within 2 hours of bedtime and being recumbent after meals is recommended. Resting LES pressure is usually normal in GERD.

Hiatal hernia is variably present in GERD, being more common in patients over 60 years of age (5), and may play a role in making esophagitis more severe due to impaired esophageal clearance. Ineffective esophageal motility (IEM)—a manometric abnormality characterized by decreased amplitude of esophageal contraction (<30 mm Hg) in greater than 30% of swallows—is the most common manometric abnormality in GERD (seen in ~35% of patients) (6,7). Patients with this motility abnormality have delayed esophageal acid clearance, creating a milieu for greater mucosal damage. Gastric acid secretion seems to be normal in patients with GERD. Studies of gastric emptying in GERD have yielded conflicting results; however, in the average patient, gastric emptying is normal. Exceptions may be seen in dyspepsia patients who experience bloating, belching, early satiety, or other motility-like symptoms.

Diagnosis

A clinical diagnosis of GERD can be made if symptoms are relieved with a therapeutic trial of antireflux therapy or by diagnostic testing with barium radiographs, esophagoscopy, or prolonged pH monitoring. When used appropriately, these tests demonstrate that reflux is occurring, identify the end-organ effects of reflux, confirm that symptoms are due to reflux, and evaluate the effects of reflux on LES pressure and esophageal clearance. The strengths and weaknesses of each study and the general guidelines for their use are reviewed below (Table 3.1).

Diagnostic Trial of Therapy

This may be the most efficient way of determining that a patient's heartburn and dyspepsia are acid mediated and due to GERD. Improvement in dyspeptic symptoms with a trial of H_2-receptor antagonists (H2RAs), prokinetic agents, or proton-pump inhibitors (PPIs) confirms that symptoms are

Table 3.1   Diagnostic Tests for Gastroesophageal Reflux and Questions Answered

Test	Questions Answered
Barium swallow	Is there a structural lesion in the patient with dysphagia?
	Is reflux or mucosal disease present (sensitivity and specificity low)?
	Is there a hiatal hernia (nonspecific finding)?
Endoscopy	Is erosive esophagitis or Barrett's esophagus present (presence of either is specific for GERD)
Ambulatory pH monitoring	Is abnormal reflux present?
	Are symptoms due to reflux?
	Is therapy optimal?
Esophageal manometry	Are motility abnormalities present that would affect surgical approach or predict outcome of treatment?

GERD = gastroesophageal reflux disease.

due to reflux. The choice of agent and the optimal length of therapeutic trial has been debated. Many clinicians favor initial treatment with H2RAs, because of decreased initial cost compared with that of PPIs. Some consider prokinetic agents for a therapeutic trial in patients who also have bloating and indigestion in addition to heartburn. Most would treat patients for 6 to 8 weeks if these agents were chosen for a trial. The literature suggests that either prescription-strength H2RAs or prokinetic agents will relieve symptoms in approximately 60% of patients (8,9). Specific studies of these agents as empirical treatment for dyspepsia suggest that either agent is superior to placebo (10,11). When reflux symptoms predominate the dyspeptic picture, PPIs are the agents of choice. Because overall symptom relief is seen in 80% to 85% of patients with GERD, these agents are preferred by some clinicians despite increased initial costs. As an empirical treatment, PPI therapy is superior to placebo for initial symptom relief, especially in the patient with reflux-type symptoms (12).

Empirical trials with high-dose (double-dose) PPIs have been suggested as a diagnostic test for GERD. One study found a sensitivity of 75% and a specificity of 55% when 1 week of omeprazole 20 mg bid was compared with endoscopy and pH monitoring (13). In another trial with ambulatory pH monitoring as the gold standard, omeprazole had a positive predictive value of 68% and negative predictive value. When omeprazole was considered the gold standard, the results were identical (14). An empirical trial of high-dose PPI has been suggested for patients with laryngitis (15) and noncardiac chest pain (16).

Patients with alarm symptoms (e.g., dysphagia, adynophagia, gastrointestinal bleeding, early satiety, weight loss, anemia) should have a diagnostic work-up to rule out complicated disease, malignancy, or both.

Barium Radiography

Barium studies are relatively inexpensive and widely available. When evaluating the esophagus for GERD, a double-contrast barium swallow should be ordered to ensure optimal evaluation. The most common findings are hiatal hernia and free reflux of barium. A hiatal hernia is seen in approximately 60% of healthy patients over 60 years of age (5). Free reflux may be seen in up to 30% of normal patients and be absent in up to 30% of patients with proven GERD by pH monitoring (17), making neither finding diagnostic. Specific mucosal abnormalities seen in patients with erosive esophagitis are seen in a minority of patients with GERD, making this study relatively insensitive for the diagnosis of esophagitis. The diagnosis of Barrett's esophagus is rarely suggested by a barium swallow.

The barium study is indicated as part of the evaluation of the patient with suspected complications of GERD (e.g., motility abnormalities, peptic stricture). These are abnormalities that should be considered in patients presenting with solid and/or liquid dysphagia—a symptom rarely seen in patients presenting with dyspepsia. An upper GI series, best used to evaluate the stomach and duodenum, has little (if any) use in the diagnosis of GERD in the patient with dyspepsia.

Endoscopy

Endoscopy is the best test to document mucosal abnormalities and to establish a diagnosis of erosive esophagitis, peptic stricture, or Barrett's esophagus. In the patient with GERD-related dyspepsia, endoscopy is most often normal; most patients have nonerosive GERD. In patients with dyspepsia, the frequency of complications (particularly Barrett's esophagus) is not known. Barrett's esophagus is present in 12% to 20% of patients undergoing endoscopy for heartburn (18,19) and is seen most commonly in white men over 50 years of age who have had GERD symptoms for more than 5 years.(20)

There are no absolute indications for endoscopy in the patient with suspected GERD. General guidelines suggest that the following individuals should be considered for endoscopy: symptomatic patients with heartburn who fail to respond to a 6- to 8-week therapeutic trial of pharmacologic therapy and patients who have symptoms for more than 3 to 5 years, are over 50 years of age, and/or have alarm symptoms (21). Guidelines for endoscopy in the patient with dyspepsia should be considered relevant for the patient with heartburn. Patients with Barrett's esophagus require periodic endoscopic screening (every 2–3 years) because of an increased risk of adenocarcinoma (18).

Esophageal Biopsy

Mucosal biopsy and cytology are of limited value in GERD patient evaluation unless Barrett's esophagus or malignancy is suspected. The light microscopic signs of GERD are relatively nonspecific and do not aid in the diagnosis. Microscopic signs of acute esophagitis are present in less than 30% of adult patients with GERD (22) and as such are insensitive diagnostic findings.

If the endoscopic appearance is suggestive of Barrett's esophagus, then a systematic biopsy protocol should be followed to confirm the diagnosis and rule out dysplasia or carcinoma (18). Endoscopic surveillance every 2 or more years with biopsy specimens taken to rule out dysplasia is the standard of practice for patients with Barrett's esophagus. Because there are no recommendations as to how long this should be continued, no definite recommendation can be made regarding at what age surveillance can end.

Prolonged Ambulatory pH Monitoring

Prolonged ambulatory pH monitoring is the best test for quantifying esophageal acid exposure and determining whether symptoms are due to GERD. The study has increased value in patients with atypical symptoms, including dyspepsia. This study is performed by placing a 2-mm diameter catheter transnasally into the distal esophagus with an electrode 5 cm above the LES, which is located by esophageal manometry. A small microcomputer is worn on a belt or clipped to the waist so that the patient can be monitored in an ambulatory setting. Activity can be tailored to provoke reflux in the setting in which symptoms are normally produced. For example, a patient who develops dyspeptic symptoms after a meal or after imbibing alcohol can be monitored with instructions to reproduce that clinical situation.

The microcomputer (data logger) has a symptom button for the patient to record up to six symptoms during the study. The patient is asked to record symptoms and meal times on a diary card. This allows correlation of reflux events with symptoms, which is especially valuable in patients who present with symptoms other than heartburn. Multiple electrodes can be placed on a single catheter to monitor intragastric and intra-esophageal pH, allowing for the assessment of gastric acid response to antisecretory therapy and of symptom correlation with esophageal acid exposure.

Prolonged pH monitoring is indicated when 1) symptoms other than heartburn are suspected to have been caused by GERD, 2) heartburn is accompanied by a negative endoscopy in patients who have failed a therapeutic trial, 3) the response to medical therapy is being assessed, and 4) a pre-operative evaluation for antireflux surgery is being obtained. Dual-channel monitoring is recommended to evaluate patients with pulmonary or laryngeal symptoms, because the finding of proximal reflux seems to predict the response to medical therapy (23,24).

Esophageal Manometry

Esophageal manometry can establish an abnormality of LES pressure or esophageal motility. Its major use in GERD is in pre-operative evaluation. The presence of esophageal motility abnormalities (principally hypotensive, disordered peristalsis [IEM]) changes the surgical approach. The surgeon will likely perform a Nissen fundoplication (360° wrap) in patients with normal peristalsis and a Toupet procedure (240° wrap) when distal esophageal motility abnormalities (IEM) are present (25).

Hiatal Hernia

The frequency of hiatal hernia findings negates its clinical importance. Few patients with a radiographically demonstrated hernia actually have heartburn, suggesting that a hiatal hernia alone has little importance as a cause of GERD.

Hernias, however, do change the relationship of the LES and crural diaphragm, displacing the LES above the diaphragm where the low pressure in the hernia sac acts as a reservoir for acid, allowing earlier reflux during LES relaxation and delaying esophageal clearance (26). Patients with large hernias who also have low LES pressure may be more prone to reflux (27), which suggests that a hiatal hernia should be viewed as a factor in contributing to the severity of the disease but not considered synonymous with GERD.

Treatment

Treating the patient with GERD requires consideration of the symptom presentation and the presence or absence of mucosal injury and complications. We look to achieve four goals: elimination of symptoms, healing of mucosal injury if present, management of complications, and maintenance of symptomatic remission. Treatment combines appropriate lifestyle modifications, pharmacologic therapy, and antireflux surgery when appropriate. GERD is a chronic disease and often will recur quickly if therapy is stopped or medication dose is decreased; therefore, long-term therapy is the key to effective management and often requires continuous full-prescription doses of appropriate medications Symptom relief and mucosal healing in GERD are related directly to the control of intragastric acid secretion (time gastric pH < 4) and reduction of esophageal acid exposure.

Clinical trials in patients with heartburn as the primary symptom suggest that a careful and systematic stepwise approach to medical therapy results in satisfactory symptom relief for almost all patients. Treatment therefore is based on clinical experience and on the principles for treating patients with heartburn and erosive esophagitis. The end points outlined above, relief of symptoms, healing of mucosal injury, and maintenance of remission, are still the primary goals; however, assessing these end points in dyspepsia patients is somewhat more difficult because the "gold standard" for diagnosis is not always clear.

Lifestyle Modification and Patient Education

Simple and effective changes in lifestyle are crucial in controlling symptoms of GERD. Patient education about the chronicity of GERD and dyspepsia is critical to achieve prolonged compliance with medical management. Studies with overnight pH monitoring have shown a significant decrease in total esophageal acid exposure after elevating the head of the bed 6 inches compared with sleeping flat (28–30). A similar effect can be produced by placing a foam rubber wedge under the patient's mattress. A long (full-length) wedge is preferable to tilt the whole mattress, rather than bending it at the waist level. Acid exposure is more frequent when the patient lies or sleeps on his or her right side compared with the left side and recumbent position (30). Based on this information, we suggest that patients sleep on their left side when possible.

Reducing esophageal irritants from the diet will help decrease symptoms. These agents include citrus juices, tomato products, coffee (both caffeinated and decaffeinated), and alcohol (beer has an acidic pH). Colas, tea, and other acidic fluids are overlooked as potential esophageal irritants (31). A meal with a high-fat content increases postprandial reflux episodes in patients with GERD (32), so a low-fat diet is recommended. Chocolate, other carminatives, and onions lower LES pressure and increase reflux frequency (33,34).

Gastric distention is the major stimulus for TLESR, the most common abnormality responsible for individual reflux episodes. Eating large, high-fat meals increases gastric distention, slows gastric emptying, and likely increases TLESR. Retiring to bed on a full stomach or lying down after a meal (particularly on the right side) is likely to increase reflux (30). This lifestyle modification (i.e., not eating within 2–3 hours of sleep and avoiding recumbency after meals) may be the most important of all.

Medications that decrease esophageal pressures and promote reflux include anticholinergics, sedatives, tranquilizers, tricyclic antidepressants, theophylline, nitrates, and calcium-channel blockers. Other drugs may cause direct esophageal injury (pill-induced esophagitis) (35); these include potassium-chloride tablets, iron sulfate, gelatin-capsule antibiotics, nonsteroidal anti-inflammatory drugs (NSAIDs), and alendronate (Fosamax). Although we have no direct evidence that these agents cause GERD, they can cause esophageal injury and may make mucosal injury from reflux more severe. However, the effects of these agents vary from patient to patient, and experience suggests that none of these drugs greatly exacerbates GERD, so discontinuing an essential drug is not necessary. Smoking decreases LES pressure and delays esophageal clearance—likely due to the direct effects of nicotine—thereby increasing reflux frequency and mucosal injury potential. Clearly, smoking can be detrimental to overall health, and the exacerbation of GERD is no exception.

The importance of lifestyle modifications as part of a treatment program when efficacious drug therapy (e.g., PPIs) is available has been debated. Because clinical trials have always included these changes as part of treatment, the effect of eliminating them has not been studied. These interventions are easy to explain and are of low economic cost. Based on symptom severity and control, patients should decide for themselves how carefully to follow them. Some patients with mild, infrequent symptoms may avoid having to take regular prescription medications by following these recommendations. The effect of lifestyle modifications on dyspepsia has not been specifically studied.

Over-the-Counter Agents

Antacids and H2RAs are used commonly in the treatment of dyspepsia and GERD. These agents are used exclusively for the treatment of intermittent symptoms and occasionally as adjuncts to prescription therapy for breakthrough symptoms. Symptom relief is similar among equipotent antacids and all over-the-counter H2RAs.

Prescription H$_2$-Receptor Antagonists

Since the late 1970s, H2RAs have been the most commonly prescribed treatment for GERD. These drugs inhibit gastric acid secretion and have no effect on LES pressure or esophageal clearance. The four available agents (cimetidine, ranitidine, famotidine, and nizatidine) have the same efficacy when used in equivalent doses (Table 3.2). These agents are extremely well tolerated in all age groups and achieve relief of heartburn in approximately 60% of patients, with maximum effects seen after 6 to 8 weeks (11). Healing of mucosal abnormalities in the esophagus is less frequent and often overestimated, being seen in 0% to 82% (mean 48%) of patients (36). The best results are seen in those with nonerosive esophagitis, suggesting that they may be useful in dyspepsia patients who have endoscopy-nega-

Table 3.2   Drugs Used in the Pharmacologic Treatment of Gastroesophageal Reflux Disease

Drug	Mechanism of Action	Recommended Dosage	Side Effects	Comments
H2RAs	Inhibit gastric acid secretion		Very safe agents; hepatitis (rarely), qualitative platelet defects, and mental confusion seen with IV use	Higher dosages (up to 4×/d) are needed to treat erosive esophagitis; exercise caution when using concurrently with dilantin, warfarin, or theophylline
Cimetidine		800 mg bid		
Ranitidine		150 mg bid-qid		
Famotidine		20 mg bid		
Nizatidine		150 mg bid		
Prokinetic agents				
Cisapride*	Increases GI motility, enhances salivary flow	10 mg qid or 20 mg bid	Diarrhea (in ~10% of patients), nausea	Cisapride has similar efficacy to that of H2RAs for GERD ECG required before use
Metoclopramide	Increases esophageal (minimally) and gastric motility and LESP	10–15 mg every half-hour AC plus qhs	Parkinson's-like tremors, somnolence, and agitation	Tachyphylaxis (warning effect) with extended use (>6 months); high side-effect profile
PPIs	Inhibit gastric acid secretion		Excellent safety profile; diarrhea (rarely) and headache	Superior to H2RAs; profound acid suppression
Omeprazole		20 mg qAM		
Lansoprazole		30 mg qAM		
Rabeprazole		20 mg qAM		
Pantoprazole		40 mg qAM		
Esomeprazole (approval anticipated)		40 mg qAM (expected dosage)		

AC = before meals; ECG = electrocardiogram, GERD = gastroesophageal reflux disease; GI = gastrointestinal; H2RAs = H$_2$-receptor antagonists; IV = intravenous; LESP = lower esophageal sphincter pressure; PPIs = proton-pump inhibitors.
* Cisapride has been taken off the market and is available only on a restricted basis by applying to the manufacturer, Janssen Pharmaceutica.

tive disease. Higher doses of H2RAs (up to four times daily) usually are needed to treat erosive esophagitis (37). However, the cost of this double-dose therapy is greater than, and therapy is not as clinically effective as, a single daily dose of a PPI.

A recent article questions the efficacy of higher doses of H2RAs on heartburn relief (38). In this study, patients with heartburn were treated empirically with ranitidine150 mg bid for 6 weeks. Nonresponders were then randomized to receive an additional 8 weeks of treatment with either 150 mg or 300 mg bid. At the end of 8 weeks, no difference in complete symptom relief (achieved in >30%) was seen between the two groups, reinforcing that little is to be gained in doubling the dose of H2RAs in the patients with acid-related symptoms (38). Maintenance of heartburn relief and healing of esophageal mucosal injury are seen in up to 50% of patients treated with continuous therapy of H2RA for 1 year (39).

H_2-receptor antagonists are remarkably safe agents. Side effects from clinical trials are rarely greater than that of placebo. Rare cases of hepatitis, qualitative platelet defects, and mental confusion have been reported with intravenous use. Drug interactions are extremely rare, although they seem to be slightly more prevalent with cimetidine. Caution should be exercised in patients on dilantin, warfarin, and theophylline, but clinical problems are rare.

Prokinetic Agents

The pathogenesis of GERD is related to defects in esophagogastric motility, LES incompetence, poor esophageal clearance, and delayed gastric emptying. Therapy directed at correcting these defects allows improvement in GERD symptoms without suppression of gastric acid. Cisapride, previously the most commonly prescribed prokinetic agent, increases gastrointestinal motility and enhances salivary flow, which provides its buffering capacity. Improvements in daytime and nocturnal heartburn have been demonstrated in up to 60% of patients taking cisapride 10 mg qid (40) and 20 mg bid (see Table 3.2) (41). Symptoms of dysmotility (e.g., postprandial bloating, fullness, early satiety, belching, regurgitation) can be reduced significantly by cisapride (42,43), as can symptom relief and healing of mild to moderate esophagitis. Cisapride and H2RAs show similar efficacy when compared head to head (44,45). However, combinations of cisapride with cimetidine or ranitidine enhance healing and symptom relief when compared with either of those H2RAs alone (46–48). The cost, efficacy, and potential side effects compared with PPIs suggest that this regimen should not be used. Cisapride 10 mg bid and 20 mg at bedtime may prevent relapse in 40% to 50% of patients, predominately those with nonerosive esophagitis (49,50).

The central nervous system side effects of metoclopramide (e.g., drowsiness, irritability, extrapyramidal effects) have drastically reduced its use, particularly in the elderly. Because cisapride does not cross the blood-brain barrier, these side effects are not seen; thus, cisapride has replaced metoclopramide as the prokinetic agent of choice. The major side effects of cisapride are diarrhea (~10%) and nausea. Prolongation of the QT interval and development of ventricular arrhythmias can be seen in patients on cisapride who are treated concomitantly with macrolide antibiotics (e.g., erythromycin) or antifungal agents (51). The use of these drugs in combination is contraindicated. New guidelines recommend giving cisapride only after attempting a course of antisecretory therapy. This drug is now available only on a restricted basis by applying to Janssen Pharmaceutica.

Proton-Pump Inhibitors

Proton-pump inhibitors inhibit the terminal step of acid secretion by blocking the H^+K^+ ATPase enzyme at the secretory caniliculi of the parietal cell. The profound acid inhibition achieved with these agents results in superior symptom relief and healing of erosive disease. PPIs are superior to both placebo and standard-dose H2RA therapy when compared head to head. A single daily dose of either omeprazole or lansoprazole will produce a 67% to 95% (mean 83%) rate of symptom relief and healing of erosive esophagitis (52,53). Trials with rabeprazole (released in late 1999) and pantoprazole (scheduled for U.S. release in mid-to-late 2000) also have demonstrated healing rates superior to placebo and H2RAs and seemed similar to omeprazole in one head-to-head trial (54–56). A trial that included over 1400 patients demonstrated similar healing rates after 8 weeks of therapy with either omeprazole 20 mg/d or lansoprazole 30 mg/d (57). Patients with severe esophagitis (grades III–IV) may have lower healing rates, leading to the need for higher doses of PPIs (58). A newer PPI, esomeprazole (the *s*-isomer of omeprazole), seems to provide superior healing than currently available PPIs. The role of esomeprazole in the management of GERD awaits further investigation. Some patients will continue to secrete acid, decreasing intragastric pH to less than 4, and experience nocturnal GERD despite twice-daily PPI (59). When continuous PPI therapy is administered over a 1-year period, complete symptom relief and healing of erosive esophagitis is seen in 80% of patients (39). Continuous therapy is significantly superior to half-dose, alternate-day or weekend therapy and to H2RAs in the long-term treatment of GERD. This effect is likely similar for all PPIs. Continuous therapy with omeprazole 20–60 mg/d has been shown to maintain complete symptom relief and healing in patients refractory to H2RAs for up to 5 years (58). Several key points are illustrated by this study; long-term remission is possible in up to 100% of patients if tailored doses of PPIs are used. Up to 30% of patients refractory to H2RAs will require more than a single daily dose of a PPI, and long-term remission can be maintained without developing tolerance. Continued follow-up of this same patient group shows continued success of omeprazole for up to 11 years.

The need for higher doses of PPIs has increased the use of combined intragastric and esophageal pH monitoring. This allows evaluation of the adequacy of acid suppression and control of reflux in patients with continued symptoms, particularly atypical symptoms such as dyspepsia (60). This technique can effectively monitor the dose of PPI therapy required for each patient.

Combination therapy with PPIs and prokinetics (prinicipally cisapride) is commonly used in clinical practice in patients who are difficult to manage. Unfortunately, few data are available about combination therapy versus increased doses of PPIs. PPIs are most effective when taken before meals (to allow the drug to be present when parietal cells are active). More effective pH control is achieved when given as split doses twice daily (before breakfast and dinner), rather than as a double dose once daily (61). The clinical importance of this has not been studied. Skipping breakfast will reduce the efficacy of the PPIs. If an H2RA is added, it should be given only at bedtime (*see* below).

Proton-pump inhibitors have an excellent safety profile, with no side effects greater than placebo seen in clinical trials. Headache and diarrhea are rare. The long-term safety of PPIs has been well demonstrated—ample gastric acid is produced in a 24-hour period to allow for normal protein digestion, to prevent bacterial overgrowth, and to maintain iron, calcium, and vitamin B_{12} absorption. The most important concern with long-term PPI use is hyperplasia of enterchromaffin-like cells (ECLs) and the development of gastric carcinoid tumors because of gastrin hypersecretion. There have been no reports of gastric carcinoid or malignancy with up to 11 years of omeprazole. Hyperplasia of ECL cells is seen in 4% or less of patients on PPIs. A recent study suggested that patients on long-term omeprazole who were infected with *Helicobacter pylori* developed atrophic gastritis (a proposed precursor of gastric adneocarcinoma) more rapidly than patients who were not infected. This finding prompted a recommendation for the screening and treatment of *H. pylori* in patients on long-term PPI therapy (62). Current guidelines have determined that there likely are insufficient data to support this recommendation (63); thus, no laboratory monitoring (serum gastrin in particular) is required for patients on long-term PPI therapy. Early data suggest that the newer agents rabeprazole and pantoprazole will be as safe as omeprazole and lansoprazole.

Antireflux Surgery

The successful use of laparoscopic fundoplication has changed the approach to surgery for GERD. Success rates of approximately 90% after 3 to 5 years with minimal complications make fundoplication attractive for some patients. The use of a short, loose, "floppy" fundoplication has markedly reduced the postoperative sequelae associated with antireflux surgery (e.g., dysphagia, "gas bloat") (63,64).

The indications for surgery for GERD are still debated. Medical failure is rare and, in itself, not an indication. Surgery should be considered for patients with documented, relatively severe GERD (e.g., those with erosive esophagitis, stricture, or Barrett's esophagus) and for patients without nonerosive GERD who require continuous high doses of PPIs for long-term symptom relief (Table 3.3). Antireflux surgery may be the preferred option in patients for whom medication is a financial burden, those who are noncompliant with their drug regimen, and in individuals who prefer a single intervention to long-term drug treatment.

A thorough pre-operative evaluation with esophageal manometry, pH monitoring, and endoscopy is critical to determine that GERD is the underlying cause of the patient's symptoms and to decide on the best surgical approach (65). A short esophagus can lead to an increased incidence of failure of surgery if not detected pre-operatively. Esophageal length is best assessed using barium swallow and endoscopy. A short esophagus should be suspected if there is a large (>5 cm) hiatal hernia, particularly if it fails to reduce in the upright position on video barium esophagraphy.

Complications are uncommon, and mortality is rare. In a recent review, four deaths occurred among 2453 patients (66). On average, complications arise in 10% to 15% of patients and tend to be minor (67). Unrecognized perforation of the esophagus or stomach is the most life-threatening sequela and is related to the surgeon's experience (68).

Relief of typical reflux symptoms (e.g., heartburn, regurgitation, dysphagia) is seen in more than 90% of patients after up to 3 years of follow-up. A conversion rate of 4.2% to open surgery, a 0.5% rate of early re-operation, and excellent to good symptomatic improvement in 91% of

---

Table 3.3   Considerations for Antireflux Surgery

- Severe gastroesophageal reflux disease

- Erosive esophagitis

- Stricture

- Barrett's esophagus

- Symptom relief achieved only the with long-term, high-dose PPI use

- Patient preference (e.g., inability to afford medication, noncompliance with drug regimen, preference for surgical option)

- Extra-esophageal complications (especially asthma)

PPI = proton-pump inhibitor.

patients are reported (69,70). Postoperative dysphagia has decreased to 3% to 5% with increasing experience and attention to technical details (71).

The laparoscopic technique is exciting, but these excellent results come from centers with extensive experience. One must evaluate the experience and results in the community before choosing surgery and considering whether a referral to a more experienced surgical center is appropriate.

Approach to the Patient with Dyspepsia

The approach to the patient with GERD is based predominantly on clinical experience. Patients with heartburn and regurgitation as the primary symptom of dyspepsia can be treated empirically with either a diagnostic trial or traditional step-care approach. If chosen, each level of therapeutic trial should last from 4 to 8 weeks before moving to the next step. Options are available at each step and should be based on cost, patient and physician familiarity with the agent, and the possibility of side effects from drug interaction. Complete relief of dyspepsia is the goal of acute therapy; maintenance therapy should be with the least costly agent that achieves continued symptom relief. A reasonable strategy in dyspepsia patients may be a trial off all therapy but with continued lifestyle modifications or consideration of intermittent therapy before initiating long-term maintenance.

I choose early diagnostic evaluation with endoscopy for patients with alarm symptoms of odynophagia, anemia, dysphagia, early satiety, weight loss, or gastrointestinal bleeding. Diagnostic evaluation of the dyspeptic without alarm symptoms usually should begin with a prolonged pH-monitoring study to assess symptom correlation with esophageal acid exposure. This can be performed while off therapy or, if the response to a therapeutic trial is incomplete, while continuing medical therapy. Continued symptoms can be correlated with the presence of esophageal acid exposure.

A careful, thoughtful approach to the patient with GERD and dyspepsia will produce a successful outcome in most patients.

Key Points

- GERD may be caused by abnormalities such as a defective antireflux barrier, abnormal esophageal clearance, altered esophageal clearance, altered esophageal mucosal resistance, and delayed gastric emptying.

- Empirical pharmacologic therapy (given for 6 to 8 weeks) is associated with an improvement in dyspeptic symptoms and may be the most efficient means of diagnosing GERD.

- Other diagnostic tests include barium studies, endoscopy, ambulatory pH monitoring, and esophageal manometry. Barium studies are indicated when complications such as peptic stricture are suspected. Endoscopy will identify erosive esophagitis, Barrett's esophagus, and peptic stricture. Ambulatory pH monitoring is used to assess symptom correlation with esophageal acid exposure.

- The goals of treatment are relief of symptoms, healing of mucosal injury, management of complications, and maintenance of remission. Because symptoms often will recur quickly if treatment is discontinued, long-term therapy is recommended for effective management.

- Continuous treatment with PPIs is effective in patients who are refractory to treatment with H2RAs. PPIs are also significantly superior to H2RAs in the long-term treatment of GERD.

REFERENCES

1. **The Gallup Organization.** *A Gallup Survey on Heartburn Across America.* Princeton, NJ: The Gallup Organization; 1968.

2. **Locke GR, Talley NJ, Fett SL, et al.** Prevalence and clinical spectrum of gastroesophageal reflux: a population-based study in Olmstead County, Minnesota. *Gastroenterology.* 1997;112:5–12.

3. **Nebel OT, Fornes MF, Castell DO.** Symptomatic gastroesophageal reflux: incidence and precipitating factors. *Dig Dis Sci.* 1976;21:953–6.

4. **Dent J, Dodds WJ, Friedman RH, et al.** Mechanism of gastroesophageal reflux in recumbent asymptomatic human subjects. *J Clin Invest.* 1980;65:256–67.

5. **Stilson W.** Hiatal hernia and gastroesophageal reflux. *Radiology.* 1969;93:1323–37.

6. **Leite LP, Johnston BT, Barrett J, et al.** Ineffective esophageal motility (IEM): the primary finding in patients with nonspecific esophageal motility disorder. *Dig Dis Sci.* 1997;42:1859–65.

7. **Fouad YM, Katz PO, Khoury R, Castell DO.** Ineffective esophageal motility: the common motility abnormality in patients with GERD-associated respiratory symptoms. *Am J Gastroenterol.* 1999;94:1464–7.

8. **Sontag S, Robinson M, McCallum RW, et al.** Ranitidine therapy for gastroesophageal reflux disease: results of a large double-blind trial. *Arch Intern Med.* 1987;147:1485–91.

9. **Tougas G, Armstrong D.** Efficacy of H_2-receptor antagonists in the treatment of gastroesophageal reflux disease and its symptoms. *Can J Gastroenterol.* 1997; 11(Suppl B):51B–4B.

10. **Veldhuyzen van Zanten, Jones M, Talley NJ.** Cisapride for treatment of nonulcer dyspepsia (NUD): a meta-analysis of randomized controlled trials. *Gastroenterology.* 1998;114:G1322.

11. **Dobrilla G, Comberlato M, Stelle A, Vallaperta P.** Drug treatment of functional dyspepsia: a meta-analysis of randomized controlled trials. *Gastroenterology.* 1989; 11:169–77.

12. **Johnsson F, Weywadt L, Sonhaug JN, et al.** One-week omeprazole treatment in the diagnosis of gastro-oesophageal reflux disease. *Scand J Gastroenterol.* 1998; 33:15–20.

13. **Schenk BE, Kuipers EJ, Klinkenberg-Knol EC, et al.** Omeprazole as a diagnostic tool in gastroesophageal reflux disease. *Am J Gastroenterol.* 1997;92:1997–2000.

14. **Wo JM, Grist WJ, Gussack G, et al.** Empiric trial of high-dose oemprazole in patients with posterior laryngitis: a prospective study. *Am J Gastroenterol.* 1997; 92:2160–5.

15. **Fass R, Fennerty MB, Ofman JJ, et al.** The clinical and economic value of omeprazole in patients with noncardiac chest pain. *Gastroenterology.* 1998;115: 42–9.

16. **Talley NJ, Meineche-Schmidt V, Pare P, et al.** Acid suppression efficacious in nonulcer dyspepsia?: double blind, randomized, controlled trial with omeprazole. *Gastroenterology.* 1998;114:G1248.

17. **Ott DJ, Wu WC, Gelfand DW.** Reflux esophagitis revisited: prospective analysis of radiologic accuracy. *Gastrointest Radiol.* 1981;6:1–7.

18. **Eisen GM, Sandler RS, Murray S, Gottfried M.** The relationship between gastroesophageal reflux disease and its complications with Barrett's esophagus. *Am J Gastroenterol.* 1997;92:27–31.

19. **Lieberman DA, Oehike M, Helfand M, and the GORGE Consortium.** Risk factors for Barrett's esophagus in community-based practice. *Am J Gastroenterol.* 1997;92:1293–7.

20. **DeVault KR, Castell DO.** Updated guidelines for the diagnosis and treatment of gastroesophageal reflux disease. *Am J Gastroenterol.* 1999;94:1434–42.

21. **Sampliner RE.** Practice guidelines on the diagnosis, surveillance, and therapy of Barrett's esophagus. *Am J Gastroenterol.* 1998;9:23–7.

22. **Ismail-Beigi F, Horton PF, Pope CE.** Histological consequences of gastroesophageal reflux: in man. *Gastroenterology.* 1998;95:903–12.

23. **Schnatz PF, Castell JA, Castell DO.** Pulmonary symptoms associated with gastroesophageal reflux: use of ambulatory pH monitoring to diagnose and to direct therapy. *Am J Gastroenterol.* 1996;91:1715–8.

24. **Harding SM, Richter JE, et al.** Asthma and gastroesophageal reflux: acid suppression therapy improves asthma outcome. *Am J Med.* 1996;100:395–405.

25. **Kauer WK, Peters JH, DeMeester TR, et al.** A tailored approach to antireflux surgery. *J Thorac Cardiovasc Surg.* 1995;170:614–7.

26. **Sloan S, Kahrilas PJ.** Impairment of esophageal emptying with hiatal hernia. *Gastroenterology.* 1991;100:596–605.

27. **Sloan S, Rademaker AW, Kahrilas PJ.** Determinants of gastroesophageal junction incompetence: hiatal hernia, lower esophageal sphincter, or both? *Ann Intern Med.* 1992;117:977–82.

28. **Stanciu C, Bennett JR.** Effects of posture on gastro-oesophageal reflux. *Digestion.* 1977:15:104–9.

29. **Johnson LF, DeMeester TR.** Evaluation of elevation of the head of the bed, bethanechol, and antacid foam tablets on gastroesophageal reflux. *Dig Dis Sci.* 1981;26:673–80.

30. **Khoury R, Mohiuddin M, Katz PO, Castell DO.** Influence of body position on nighttime recumbent reflux in patients with GERD. *Gastroenterology.* 1998;114:713.

31. **Wendl B, Pfeiffer A, Phel C, et al.** Effect of decaffeination of coffee or tea on gastro-oesophageal reflux. *Aliment Pharmacol Ther.* 1994;8:283–7.

32. **Becker DJ, Sinclair J, Castell DO, et al.** A comparison of high- and low-fat meals on postprandial esophageal acid exposure. *Am J Gastroenterol.* 1989;84:1076–8.

33. **Murphy DW, Castell DO.** Chocolate and heartburn: evidence of increased esophageal acid exposure after chocolate ingestion. *Am J Gastroenterol.* 1988; 83:633–6.

34. **Allen ML, Mellow MH, Robinson MG, et al.** The effect of raw onions on acid reflux and reflux symptoms. *Am J Gastroenterol.* 1990;85:377–80.

35. **Kikendall JW.** Pill-induced esophageal injury: case reports and review of the medical literature. *Dig Dis Sci.* 1983;28:174–85.

36. **Sontag S, Robinson M, McCallum RW, et al.** Ranitidine therapy for gastroesophageal reflux disease: results of a large double-blind trial. *Arch Intern Med.* 1987;147:1485–91.

37. **Euler AR, Murdock RH, Wilson TH, et al.** Ranitidine is effective therapy for erosive esophagitis. *Am J Gastroenterol.* 1993;88:520–4.

38. **Kahrilas PJ, Fennerty MB, Joelsson B.** High- versus standard-dose ranitidine for control of heartburn in poorly responsive acid reflux disease: a prospective controlled trial. *Am J Gastroenterol.* 1999;94:92–7.

39. **Vignieri S, Termini R, Leandro G, et al.** A comparison of five maintenance therapies for reflux esophagitis *N Engl J Med.* 1995;333:1106–10.

40. **Galmiche JP, Fraitag B, Filoche B, et al.** Double-blind comparison of cisapride and cimetidine in treatment of reflux esophagitis. *Dig Dis Sci.* 1990;35:649–55.

41. **Castell D, Sigmund C, Patterson D, et al.** Cisapride 20 mg bid provides effective daytime and nighttime relief in patients with symptoms of chronic gastroesophageal reflux disease. *Gastroenterology.* 1997;112:A84.

42. **Robertson CS, Evans DF, Ledingham SJ, Atkinson M.** Cisapride in the treatment of gastro-oesophageal reflux disease. *Aliment Pharmacol Ther.* 1993;7: 181–90.

43. **Tytgat GNJ, Anker Hansen OJ, Carling L, et al.** Effect of cisapride on relapse of reflux oesophagitis, healed with an antisecretory drug. *Scan J Gastroenterol.* 1992;27:175–83.

44. **Janisch HD, Huttermann W, Bouzo MH.** Cisapride versus ranitidine in the treatment of reflux esophagitis. *Hepatogastroenterology.* 1988;35:125–7.

45. **Galmiche JP, Fraitag B, Filoche B, et al.** Double-blind comparison of cisapride and cimetidine in the treatment of reflux esophagitis. *Dig Dis Sci.* 1990;35:649–55.

46. **Galmiche JP, Brandstatter G, Evreux M, et al.** Combined therapy with cisapride and cimetidine in severe reflux oesophagitis: a double-blind controlled trial. *Gut.* 1988;29:675–81.

47. **Inauen W, Emde C, Weber B, et al.** Effects of ranitidine and cisapride on acid reflux and oesophageal motility in patients with reflux oesphagitis: a 24-hour ambulatory combined pH and manometry study. *Gut.* 1993;34:1025–31.

48. **McKenna CJ, Mills JG, Goodwin C, Wood JR.** Combination of ranitidine and cisapride in the treatment of reflux oesophagitis. *Eur J Gastroenterol Hepatol.* 1995;7:817–22.

49. **Toussaint J, Gossuin A, Deruyttere M, et al.** Healing and prevention of relapse of reflux oesphagitis by cisapride. *Gut.* 1991;32:1280–5.

50. **Blum AL, Adami B, Bouzo MH, et al.** Effect of cisapride on relapse of esophagitis: a multinational, placebo-controlled trial in patients healed with an antisecretory drug. *Dig Dis Sci.* 1993;38:551–60.

51. **Chan-Tompkins NH, Babinchak TJ.** Cardiac arrhythmias associated with coadminstration of azole compounds and cisapride. *Clin Infect Dis.* 1997;24:1285.

52. **Hallerback B, Unge P, Carling L, et al.**. Omeprazole or ranitidine in long-term treatment of reflux oesophagitis. *Gastroenterology.* 1994;107:1305–11.

53. **Klinkenberg-Knol EC, Jansen JM, Festen HP, et al.** Double-blind multicentre comparison of omeprazole and ranitidine in the treatment of reflux oesphagitis. *Lancet.* 1987;1:349–51.

54. **Dekkers C, Beker PM, Thjodleifsson JA, et al. and the European Rabeprazole Study Group.** Double-blind, placebo-controlled comparison of rabeprazole 20 mg vs. omeprazole 20 mg in the treatment of erosive or ulcerative gastro-oesophageal reflux disease. *Aliment Pharmacol Ther.* 1999;13:49–57.

55. **Cloud ML, Humphries TJ.** Rabeprazole in treatment of acid peptic diseases: results of three placebo-controlled, dose-response clinical trials in duodenal ulcer, gastric ulcer, and gastroesophageal reflux disease (GERD). *Dig Dis Sci.* 1998:43:993–1000.

56. **Mossner J, Holscher AH, Herz R, et al.** A double-blind study of pantoprazole and omeprazole in the treatment of reflux oesophagitis: a multicentre trial. *Aliment Pharmacol Ther.* 1995;9:321–6.

57. **Castell DO, Richter JE, Robinson M, et al.** Efficacy and safety of lansoprazole in the treatment of erosive reflux esophagitis. *Am J Gastroenterol.* 1996;91:1749–57.

58. **Klinkenberg-Knol E, Festen H, Jansen J, et al.** Long-term treatment with omeprazole for refractory esophagitis. *Ann Intern Med.* 1994;121:161–7.

59. **Peghini PL, Katz PO, Bracy NA, Castell DO.** Nocturnal recovery of gastric acid secretion on twice-daily dosing of proton pump inhibitors. *Am J Gastroenterol.* 1998;93:763–7.

60. **Klinkenberg-Knol EC, Meuwissen SG.** Combined gastric and oesophageal pH-metry in patients with reflux disease resistant to omeprazole. *Aliment Pharmacol Ther.* 1990;4:485–9.

61. **Kuo B, Castell DO.** Optimal dosing of omeprazole 40 mg daily: effects on gastric and esophageal pH and serum gastrin in healthy controls. *Am J Gastroenterol.* 1996;91:1532–8.

62. **Kuipers EJ, Lundell L, Klinkenberg-Knol EC, et al.** Atrophic gastritis and *Helicobacter pylori* infection in patients with reflux esophagitis treated with omeprazole or fundoplication. *N Engl J Med.* 1996;334:1018–22.

63. **Howden CW, Hunt RH.** Guidelines for the management of *Helicobacter pylori* infection. *Am J Gastroenterology.* 1998;93:2330–8.

64. **Donahue PE, Samelson S, Nyhus LM, Bombeck CT.** The floppy Nissen fundoplication: effective long-term control of pathologic gastroesophageal reflux. *Arch Surg.* 1985;120:663–8.

65. **DeMeester TR, Bonavina L, Albertucci M.** Nissen fundoplication for gastroesophageal reflux disease: evaluation of primary repair in 100 consecutive patients. *Ann Surg.* 1986;204:9–20.

66. **Waring JP, Hunter JG, Oddsdottir M, et al.** The preoperative evaluation of patients considered for laparoscopic antireflux surgery. *Am J Gastroenterol.* 1995; 90:35–8.

67. **Perdikis G, Hinder RA, Lund RJ, et al.** Laparoscopic Nissen fundoplication: Where do we stand? *Surg Laparosc Endosc.* 1997;7:17–21.

68. **Urschel JD.** Complications of antireflux surgery. *Am J Surg.* 1993;166:68–70.

69. **Schauer PR, Meyers WC, Eubanks S, et al.** Mechanisms of gastric and esophageal perforations during laparoscopic Nissen fundoplication. *Ann Surg.* 1996;223:43–52.

70. **Hinder RA, Filip CJ, Wetscher G, et al.** Laparoscopic Nissen fundoplication is an effective treatment for gastroesophageal reflux disease. *Ann Surg.* 1994;220: 472–83.

71. **Jamieson GG, Watson DI, Britten-Jones R, et al.** Laparoscopic Nissen fundoplication. *Ann Surg.* 1994;220:137–45.

4

Helicobacter pylori and Nonulcer Dyspepsia

Hartley Cohen, MD

Loren Laine, MD

I f a specific diagnosis could account for the symptoms in the vast majority of people who seek care for their dyspepsia, there would be little controversy or difficulty in managing them. Unfortunately, the opposite is true; most patients who complain of dyspepsia do not have peptic ulcer disease (PUD), gastric cancer, or any other structural or biochemical abnormalities on diagnostic evaluation. Moreover, medication intolerance often cannot be blamed, and although approximately half of the study populations with unexplained dyspepsia may be shown to have a variety of putative, pathophysiologic derangements (e.g., motor function abnormalities of the stomach, gastric acid hypersecretion, heightened visceral perception), none of these factors has been documented conclusively to correlate with the nature or severity of the symptoms. Thus, for most patients, we have an insufficient understanding of the causes of their dyspepsia and, perhaps even more unfortunately, no specific or generally effective therapies.

Definition of Nonulcer Dyspepsia

Endoscopy is the standard for evaluating patients with dyspepsia (1). This is because mucosal lesions are detected more reliably by endoscopic examination than by routine barium upper gastrointestinal series. Endoscopy, however, fails to reveal a structural lesion that might explain the symptoms in approximately two thirds of patients. These patients are given a diagnosis of "nonulcer" dyspepsia (NUD). Synonyms include "functional," "nonorganic," "idiopathic," and "essential" dyspepsia. Thus, although dyspepsia represents uninvestigated symptoms, NUD indicates a diagnosis of exclusion made after a full diagnostic evaluation, including upper endoscopy, that reveals no cause for the symptoms.

Problems Using the Same Treatment Approach for Nonulcer Dyspepsia and Peptic Ulcer Disease

When considering appropriate therapy, clinicians must keep in mind the distinction between uninvestigated dyspepsia and NUD. Because approximately 15% to 20% of patients with uninvestigated dyspepsia may harbor a peptic ulcer, it may be reasonable to treat these patients with regimens directed against peptic ulcers, providing a benefit for at least that subset of PUD patients. However, once a diagnostic evaluation has been undertaken and a diagnosis of NUD has been made, it is more difficult to justify treatment with anti-ulcer therapy, because most patients with the diagnosis of NUD do not have long-term resolution of symptoms after therapy directed against PUD.

Seasoned clinicians may well ask whether the act of not treating NUD patients similarly to PUD patients is too "purist" or "academic." After all, there is the well-advocated concept that one should treat the whole patient, not simply look for the hole *in* the patient. Indeed, as with duodenal ulcer disease, there is a long-standing view that gastric acid is important in the pathogenesis of NUD. However, although acid secretory studies may be abnormal in a subset of patients with NUD (2), this is an inconsistent finding. Moreover, the concept of "Moynihan's disease"—a spectrum of dyspepsia patients that encompasses both those with ulcer craters and those with NUD—is not clinically useful because these patients are heterogeneous, do not share pathophysiologic abnormalities, and perhaps most relevantly do not similarly and reliably respond to acid suppressive therapy. *Helicobacter pylori* has been clearly established as a causative agent in patients with duodenal and gastric ulcer; when either of these ulcer types is found on endoscopic examination and *H. pylori* infection can be documented, treatment for *H. pylori* is indicated and, if effective, results in ulcer care (Table 4.1).

Helicobacter pylori and Nonulcer Dyspepsia

The discovery of *H. pylori* was a major advance in medicine. We now know that *H. pylori* is the causative agent for gastritis (histologic inflamma-

Table 4.1   Therapeutic Options for Eradicating *Helicobacter pylori*

Regimen	Drugs	Dosage	Duration
Dual therapy	Omeprazole and	40 mg qd	2 weeks
	Clarithromycin	500 mg tid	2 weeks
	or		
	RBC and	400 mg bid	4 weeks
	Clarithromycin	500 mg tid	2 weeks
Bismuth-based triple therapy	Bismuth subsalicylate,	2 tablets qid	2 weeks
	Metronidazole, and	250 mg qid	2 weeks
	Tetracycline or	500 mg qid	2 weeks
	Amoxicillin	500 mg qid	2 weeks
PPI-based triple therapy (PPI plus two antibiotics)	PPI,	PPI bid	10–14 days
	Clarithromycin, and	500 mg bid	10–14 days
	Metronidazole or	500 mg bid	10–14 days
	Amoxicillin	1000 mg bid	10–14 days
Quadruple therapy	Bismuth-based triple therapy and	*See* dosage above	2 weeks
	PPI	PPI bid	2 weeks

PPI = proton-pump inhibitor; RBC = ranitidine and bismuth citrate.

tion of the gastric mucosa) and for most cases of peptic ulcers (although acid is also necessary) and gastric low-grade MALT (mucosa-associated lymphoid tissue) lymphoma and seems to be a predisposing factor in the development of gastric carcinoma. Not surprisingly, many clinicians also sought to use *H. pylori* to explain the dilemma of NUD.

Even at first glance, however, attempts to incriminate *H. pylori* in most cases of NUD were doomed to failure because of data that were well known even before the discovery of *H. pylori*. Histologic inflammation of the gastric mucosa of many patients has been a well-recognized phenomenon for many decades, predating knowledge of *H. pylori*. Some patients with unexplained dyspepsia had this inflammation ("gastritis"), but many did not. Thus, the association between gastritis and dyspepsia was known to be inconsistent and became a controversial topic long before *H. pylori* was discovered. Severely hampering progress was a lack of treatment for reversing the gastritis; thus, the hypothesis that there was a causative relationship between gastritis and NUD—even if only in an unidentified subgroup of patients—could not be adequately tested.

Hypotheses Linking *Helicobacter pylori* and Nonulcer Dyspepsia

With the discovery that *H. pylori* was the cause for nearly all cases of gastritis and that gastritis resolves after cure of *H. pylori* infection, the relationship between *H. pylori*, its associated gastritis, and NUD became a subject of much investigation. However, most of the studies were of poor quality, dubious validity, and limited ability to be generalized in addition to being contradictory and confusing. Proposed hypotheses that support an etiologic role for *H. pylori* in NUD include the following:

1. The prevalence of *H. pylori* is increased in dyspepsia patients compared with asymptomatic individuals.

2. Specific symptoms are linked to *H. pylori* infection.

3. NUD-related pathophysiologic abnormalities (e.g., in gastric motor function or acid secretion) are caused by *H. pylori*.

4. An amelioration of symptoms occurs after *H. pylori* eradication.

Available data both support and refute these hypotheses, which is why the nature of the possible association between *H. pylori* and NUD is controversial. In this review, we do not attempt to detail the literature; however, we have relied on selected studies that are considered to be better designed to provide a concise appreciation of the "state of the art" of these topics and to give the reader bottom-line conclusions.

Prevalence of *Helicobacter pylori* and Nonulcer Dyspepsia

In 1996, a meta-analysis found that the prevalence of *H. pylori* infection in patients with NUD was approximately twice that of controls (3); however, many of the studies in this meta-analysis were not necessarily designed to assess this relationship. Some studies did not specifically exclude patients with a past history of ulcers. Moreover, the prevalence of *H. pylori* varied considerably depending on age, socioeconomic status, ethnicity, and geographic location, and many of the studies did not control for these variables. Thus, it is unwise to accept the findings of this meta-analysis at face value. Furthermore, even if there is an increased prevalence of *H. pylori* infection in patients with NUD, it would still be necessary to show that this reflects more than a chance occurrence of two common events. In better-designed studies, after excluding patients with PUD, the prevalence of *H. pylori* infection in patients with dyspepsia was similar to the control cohort population, approximately 30% to 50% in developed countries (4–7). In developing countries, demonstrating an increased association between *H. pylori* and various disorders versus controls might be more difficult because the background prevalence of *H. pylori* infection is high. Therefore it is not surprising that in India there is a similar prevalence of *H. pylori* infection among asymptomatic (76%) and dyspeptic (78%) individuals (8). However, a study from Saudi Arabia showed that *H. pylori* was significantly more common in asymptomatic individuals (80%) than in dyspeptics (65%) (9). Thus, patients with NUD have not been clearly documented to have an increased prevalence of *H. pylori* infection.

Association of *Helicobacter pylori* and Symptoms in Nonulcer Dyspepsia

Nonulcer dyspepsia has been categorized according to the dominant symptom complex present, i.e., "ulcer-like," "dysmotility-like," "reflux-like," and "unspecified." The characteristics of these different symptom profiles are deliberately not described herein (but may be appreciated intuitively) because most patients have symptoms that overlap, are not predictive of pathology on endoscopy, or may vary over time, resulting in unpredictable responsiveness to therapy. Nonetheless, studies both support and refute the contention that specific symptoms are caused by *H. pylori* infection. In one study, a greater improvement in ulcer-like symptoms compared with other profiles was found after *H. pylori*-infected dyspepsia patients were cured (10). However, the number of patients in this subgroup was not reported, and it is difficult to interpret the results of this study. Moreover, in this study, 14% percent of patients with persistent *H. pylori* infection developed peptic ulcers; in retrospect, they did not have NUD. It is possible that the reduction in ulcer-like symptoms was due to unrecognized PUD being cured in those who had been cured of their *H. pylori* infection. In any event, carefully performed prevalence studies did not support an association between a specific symptom profile and *H. pylori* infection (4,5).

Helicobacter pylori and Pathophysiologic Disorders in Nonulcer Dyspepsia

First, there is only a rudimentary understanding of the pathophysiologic associations between *H. pylori* and NUD. Moreover, it is uncertain if abnormalities observed bear any relation to symptoms. Second, whether *H. pylori* causes any of these abnormalities has not been studied extensively. However, the reader will note that a recurrent theme of this review is that there are contradictory and confusing data. Thus, the reader will not be surprised that accelerated, delayed, and normal gastric motor functions have been observed in dyspepsia patients with *H. pylori* infection, although a dominant relationship has not emerged (11–14). The conflicting results no doubt reflect the heterogeneous nature of NUD, and the absence of any dominant relationship between *H. pylori* and gastroduodenal motility highlights the uncertain and dubious role of *H. pylori* as a causative factor in either motor abnormalities or NUD symptoms.

Other investigators have evaluated the relationship between gastric acid secretion, *H. pylori* infection, and NUD (2,15,16). Again, the data are conflicting, and any such relationship is unconvincing even in the study that supports it. This latter study (2) found that, in patients with NUD and *H. pylori* infection, acid secretion (in response to gastrin-releasing peptide) fell among patients with duodenal ulcers and asymptomatic volunteers infected with *H. pylori*. The authors concluded that approximately 50% of

NUD patients had stimulated acid outputs similar to that of patients with duodenal ulcer disease.

One of the more interesting pathophysiologic processes in NUD is the phenomenon of augmented visceral perception in NUD patients. For example, patients with NUD report pain during intragastric balloon inflation at significantly lower levels than that tolerated by normal subjects. There is no substantive evidence, however, linking a heightened sensitivity to pain to *H. pylori* infection (17,18).

Treatment Outcomes in Clinical Trials

The recognition that *H. pylori* is responsible for nearly all chronic active and chronic superficial gastritis removed the major stumbling block of the pre-*H. pylori* era—namely, the inability to reverse or cure this gastritis and re-evaluate dyspepsia patients. After cure of the infection with antibiotics, the acute histologic inflammatory infiltrate in the gastric mucosa that is characteristic of *H. pylori* infection was found to resolve usually within a few weeks, whereas the chronic inflammatory changes improved more slowly, over months and possibly years. Thus, it became possible to test directly the hypothesis that *H. pylori* infection and its associated gastritis are responsible for dyspeptic symptoms.

A number of short-term (usually 1- to 2-month) trials were conducted in dyspeptic patients infected with *H. pylori*. In most of the earlier trials, patients were given only suppressive therapy (consisting mainly of bismuth compounds that only temporarily cleared up *H. pylori* infection), but some studies used curative therapy. Symptoms were assessed before and after treatment using a variety of symptom-scoring methods that accounted for the wide variety and variable symptoms of the study population. Although in approximately half of the studies mean symptom scores improved more in patients receiving active treatment than in controls, the remainder of the studies demonstrated that symptoms improved similarly among participants whether they received active treatment or placebo and whether their infection was successfully cured or they were uninfected controls. In most of these trials anti-*H. pylori* therapy was not adequately blinded, symptom improvement was a nebulous end point based on scoring systems that had not been validated, follow-up was short, curative anti-*H. pylori* therapies were not used, and few uninfected controls were treated. More recent randomized treatment trials used curative therapy and had follow-up periods of 6 months to 1 year (10,19,20). In two of these trials (19,20), fewer than 50 patients each were enrolled, but the treatment of *H. pylori* was associated with a progressive decline in symptoms over the follow-up duration. In the other study (10)—referred to earlier in this chapter—100 patients were randomized to receive either bismuth-based triple therapy or bismuth alone. Those who became *H. pylori* negative had a significant improvement in their symptom score at 6 months without additional improvement at 1 year. However, when the symptoms were categorized, improvement in scores was apparent for the group of patients with reflux-like and motility-like symptoms at 6 months (similarly, no improvement was seen at 1 year). Moreover, among patients in the nonspecific dyspepsia group, there was no improvement in the symptom scores at any time. This varied nature of symptomatic improvement casts doubt on the applicability of the findings to clinical practice. Furthermore, the center at which this trial was conducted also participated in a multicenter trial that is reviewed below, in which no benefit of *H. pylori* treatment was noted (21). The overall conclusions to be drawn from these trials are that there are many methodologic flaws in these studies, that the results are conflicting at best, that any improvement observed is marginal, that there is a significant response to placebo (~25%), and that routine anti-*H. pylori* therapy is not warranted for patients who present with NUD.

Two recently published, well-done studies that partially address some of the shortcomings of earlier trials deserve particular attention (21,22). These trials had large sample sizes (n = ~300 for each), used curative anti-*H. pylori* therapy that did not contain bismuth (bismuth makes blinding nearly impossible), were double-blinded and placebo-controlled, and had follow-up periods of 1 year; however, only patients infected with *H. pylori* were studied.

Because there are important differences between these trials that may influence our thinking about NUD and *H. pylori* infection, it is worthwhile to review them in detail.

The Multinational Study

One of the trials (21) was a multinational study in which over 300 *H. pylori*-infected patients were enrolled. Patients were eligible for inclusion even if they had up to five gastric erosions detected on upper endoscopy. However, patients were ineligible if they had esophageal or duodenal erosions, a history of PUD, or reflux esophagitis or heartburn as a component of their dyspepsia symptoms. Indeed, "only patients with moderate or severe pain or discomfort centered in the upper abdomen" were enrolled, suggesting that the results of this study may not be able to be generalized to most patients with NUD. Patients were randomized to receive 1 week of omeprazole (a proton-pump inhibitor) plus two antibiotics or omeprazole plus placebo. *H. pylori* was cured in approximately 80% of the patients given antibiotics. Treatment success (defined as having no symptoms or no more than minimal pain or discomfort during any of the 7 days before the 12-month follow-up visit) was 28% in those receiving antibiotics and 21% in those receiving placebo, a nonsignificant difference. Furthermore, in the group given antibiotics, treatment success was similar whether or not *H. pylori* was successfully cured. Of note, the study design called for a repeat endoscopy at 12 months, and this may have reassured participants that they had no serious illness, thus potentially augmenting a placebo response. Peptic ulcers developed in seven patients, all but one of whom had persistent *H. pylori* infection. At 1 year, histologic gastritis had resolved in only approximately 80% of patients in whom *H. pylori* was cured.

The Scottish Study

The other trial (22) was a single-center Scottish study in which more than 300 patients were randomized to receive a 2-week course of either omeprazole and antibiotics or omeprazole and placebo (22). Patients with heartburn were included in the study. Although the predominant symptom was epigastric pain, nearly half of the patients had retrosternal pain, reflux, or other unspecified symptoms as their main complaint. At 1-year follow-up, dyspeptic symptoms during the preceding 6 months were assessed. In contrast to the multicenter study, endoscopy was not performed except at entry into the study. Eighty-eight percent of patients treated with antibiotics had a negative urea breath test at follow-up. The mean dyspepsia score at 1 year follow-up was not significantly different between the two groups, but 21% of patients treated with antibiotics were free of symptoms compared with 7% of dyspepsia patients treated with omeprazole alone ($p <$ 0.001). The predominant symptom on presentation was not found to be predictive of response. Curiously, the longer the history of dyspepsia, the less likely was the resolution of symptoms with cure of *H. pylori* infection. Four patients in the omeprazole-only group were found to have ulcers when a follow-up endoscopy was performed on those with persistent symptoms.

Comparison of the Multinational and Scottish Studies

In one important respect, the treatment outcomes of the two studies were similar: 20% to 30% of patients responded to antibiotic treatment. However, the remarkable finding in the Scottish study is the low placebo-response rate of only 7% (22). There are insufficient data to explain the poor placebo-response rate in Scotland. One may speculate that many more Scottish patients in the omeprazole-only arm developed peptic ulcers compared with patients in the multicenter study in which the number of ulcers that developed was known (<3%). Inclusion criteria were different for the two studies: the Scottish study did not exclude patients with heartburn, although it is uncertain how this may have influenced the results. Successful outcome was defined as the absence of symptoms for 6 months before follow-up in the Scottish study. Conceivably, a larger proportion of patients in the omeprazole-only group may have been asymptomatic if the time frame for symptom assessment had been similar to the multicenter study (only 1 week before follow-up). In the multicenter study, at the 12-month follow-up endoscopic examination, 10 patients who had been given antibiotics were found to have erosive esophagitis compared with only three patients treated with placebo. The development of new lesions, possibly associated with symptoms (no data were given in the report) may have obfuscated a benefit of *H. pylori* treatment in the multicenter study. Because endoscopy was not performed routinely in the Scottish study, similar data are not available for comparison. Although the two studies arrive at contradictory results (epitomizing all preceding literature on this topic), it is important not to lose sight of the consistencies between them (e.g., three fourths of patients with NUD are not "cured" with anti-*H. pylori* treatment). Moreover, it is not possible to characterize which patients might respond, although response in the Scottish study was less likely in patients with a longer history of dyspepsia. Interestingly, in the multicenter study, gastritis did not resolve by 1 year in all patients who were successfully cured of *H. pylori* infection. Whether this will occur with a longer follow-up is not known, but if so it is not known whether symptoms will improve in parallel. An intriguing post hoc analysis of posttreatment gastritis scores at 1 year in a different multicenter study (23) of virtually the same design as the one reviewed above showed greater symptom improvement in those in whom gastritis had resolved. However, the main result of this other multicenter study confirms the lack of a benefit for anti-*H. pylori* treatment in NUD patients. Furthermore, because none of these studies enrolled non–*H. pylori*-infected patients, the specificity of any beneficial effect of anti-*H. pylori* therapy, especially in the Scottish study, is uncertain.

Management of Nonulcer Dyspepsia

Management of patients with NUD is problematic. In this (or any other) group, clinicians should not test for *H. pylori* unless they are prepared to treat the infection if the test is positive. Thus, for patients who have been diagnosed with NUD and are positive for *H. pylori* infection, the answer to the question of whether to treat with antibiotics is simply "Yes."

A more difficult question is, "*Should* patients diagnosed with NUD be tested for *H. pylori* infection?" The down side to *H. pylori* treatment is the possibility of increasing the rate of resistant bacteria, the potential for serious side effects (e.g., pseudomembranous colitis, which fortunately is rare), the high probability that therapy will not prove beneficial, and the possibility of inducing reflux esophagitis. However, our view is that the potential benefits of treatment may be justified because they outweigh these concerns. These potential benefits include 1) ulcer prevention in patients destined to develop them, 2) hypothetical reduction in gastric cancer risk, and 3) symptom improvement in a subset of dyspepsia patients (even though we cannot define this subset of likely responders, and treatment outcomes may represent only a placebo effect).

However, it should not be inferred that we favor anti-*H. pylori* treatment in this setting. We do not advocate or encourage such treatment because most patients will fail to respond, which may lead to fruitless testing for *H. pylori* to confirm a cure. A vicious cycle of test, treat, retest, and retreat may ensue, with a misplaced fixation on the "importance" of *H. pylori* that undermines other considerations. However, if patients request *H. pylori* testing and treatment, we are willing to comply after explaining our skepticism about the efficacy of such an approach. Moreover, a common sense approach to the treatment of NUD remains a cornerstone in our practice. It may require some sleuthing to unearth the various ingestible triggers of dyspepsia (e.g., despite direct questioning, some patients who self-medicate with aspirin, nonsteroidal anti-inflammatory agents, iron compounds, or other substances initially deny such use), but the identification and incrimination of such factors is rewarding for both physician and patient. We also often resort to administering antidepressants, usually beginning with a low dose (e.g., amitriptyline 10 µg, escalating the dose by 10 µg weekly up to 50 mg/d in the absence of a response). Although there is little evidence in support of such therapy in NUD, benefit has been demonstrated in other functional disorders, such as unexplained chest pain and irritable bowel syndrome. Treatment of *H. pylori* should not preclude these other modalities.

Management of Dyspepsia Patients with Alarm Features

How should the studies reviewed earlier influence management of patients with dyspepsia (i.e., "uninvestigated" dyspepsia)? The question is not easily answered because patients present in a variety of ways. Some patients may have "alarm" symptoms or signs (e.g., weight loss, vomiting, occult or overt blood loss from the gastrointestinal tract, anemia). The greatest concern is that a patient with such features may have an upper gastrointestinal tract malignancy. The prevalence of malignancy in dyspepsia patients with alarm symptoms is not known. Even if a patient does have gastric cancer, it is doubtful whether an immediate evaluation (usually by endoscopy) affects the poor long-term outcome in a patient presenting with symptomatic gastric carcinoma; a 1- or 2-month delay is also unlikely to affect outcome. Hence, one might argue that little would be lost by instituting initial empirical treatment even for the group of patients presenting with alarm symptoms. Nonetheless, current dogma dictates that patients with *any* alarm sign or symptom should undergo prompt diagnostic evaluation to exclude structural lesions (e.g., malignancy, ulcers causing bleeding or obstruction) rather than initially being treated empirically.

Management of Dyspeptic Patients Without Alarm Features

Most patients without alarm symptoms who present with dyspepsia will have no organic cause of their symptoms identified. PUD and reflux esophagitis may be present in 20% to 30%. Gastric cancer occurs infrequently in this setting (<3% in Western countries) but probably varies depending on the age, ethnic background, and geographic location of patients, among other factors.

Based on assumptions about costs, recurrence of symptoms, and underlying diagnoses, one decision analysis suggested that there is little to be gained by not performing endoscopy initially (26), the benefits of which may be summarized as follows: 1) there is no need for specialist evaluation, 2) a few patients will be spared the monetary cost of the procedure, and 3) some patients will avoid the minimal risk of endoscopy. Two decision analyses suggest that testing for *H. pylori* and treating those who are positive with anti-*H. pylori* therapy (the "test and treat" strategy) is a cost-effective approach (23,24). The assumptions behind this approach include that 80% of those with ulcers will be cured, that there also will be a placebo-response rate of 20% to 40% (unless the patient is from Glasgow!), and that the costs of endoscopy will be saved (even if only for a minority of patients, because endoscopy is still recommended for those in whom symptoms persist or recur). Economic models do indicate, however, that if the cost of endoscopy is low and the rate of recurrent symptoms after *H. pylori* therapy is high, initial endoscopy does become the dominant strategy instead of an initial "test and treat" strategy (24). Disadvantages of initial "test and treat" strategy include the following (27):

1. Because no more than 20% of patients with *H. pylori* infection will have ulcer disease, it is necessary to treat at least five persons for one of them to benefit.

2. There will be an incidence, however minimal, of serious side effects related to antibiotic treatment.

3. Resistance to antibiotics will be promoted.

4. Most patients will still require endoscopy (albeit delayed) for persistent symptoms.

5. Some patients may develop reflux esophagitis as a result of *H. pylori* eradication, mitigating any potential benefit of treatment.

6. By not initially performing endoscopy, the reassurance that there is no serious illness (which could result in less health care seeking behavior) may be lost.

We believe that a "test and treat" strategy is an acceptable approach pending clinical studies to evaluate whether cost savings are confirmed.

Summary

H. pylori has not been established to cause NUD. Treatment trials of *H. pylori* have yielded conflicting and confusing results, but symptoms resolve in no more than 20% to 30% of patients at best. One elegant study concluded that there was a clear beneficial response to anti-*H. pylori* treatment, but this was because the placebo-response rate was only 7% (22). Most other studies have placebo response rates similar to active therapy (e.g., anti-*H. pylori* treatment, acid suppressive therapy, other therapy) (28). In contrast with a consensus group's recommendations (29), our view is that *H. pylori* treatment should not be advocated for patients with NUD. We look forward to a better understanding of this entity and await more effective treatment. We think that testing for *H. pylori* in nonulcer dyspepsia patients and treating those who are positive is acceptable, but in our practice we restrict such an approach to those who request it.

However, we do think that the use of a "test and treat" strategy in patients with dyspepsia is reasonable, based primarily on economic modeling. Patients presenting with dyspepsia (especially those without alarm symptoms) undergo *H. pylori* testing with simple and inexpensive antibody testing (with treatment provided to those who test positive). Most of these patients will have recurrent symptoms, because only 20% or less will have ulcer disease, leaving the majority with NUD or reflux disease who will not experience a resolution of their symptoms after anti-*H. pylori* therapy. Nevertheless, by avoiding endoscopy in even a small number of patients, costs should decrease without increasing clinical risk significantly.

Recommendations

- In patients presenting with uninvestigated dyspepsia, perform *H. pylori* testing and, if results are positive, give anti-*H. pylori* treatment with a 2-week course of triple therapy (e.g., proton-pump inhibitor plus clarithromycin 500 mg bid and amoxicillin 1 g bid or metronidazole 500 mg bid for 14 days). If results are negative, proceed with diagnostic evaluation (typically including endoscopy), with direct testing toward the cause (e.g., ulcer-like [endoscopy] vs. motility-like [gastric emptying studies]). We believe that this "test and treat" strategy is an acceptable initial management option, except when endoscopy is indicated at presentation (i.e., in patients with alarm symptoms [e.g., weight loss, vomiting, bleeding, dysphagia]).

- Based on our clinical experience, *H. pylori* testing is not indicated and anti-*H. pylori* treatment is not sufficiently effective in patients diagnosed with NUD. However, *H. pylori* testing should be given to those NUD patients who request it and treatment should be provided for those in whom test results are positive.

Key Points

- With the discovery of *H. pylori* as the cause of most cases of PUD, recent attempts have been made to find a similar association between NUD and *H. pylori* infection.

- Studies both support and refute the proposal that specific symptoms are linked to *H. pylori* infection. Similarly, studies evaluating the pathophysiologic abnormalities of NUD have offered conflicting results.

- Studies evaluating anti-*H. pylori* treatment in patients with NUD have yielded confusing and contradictory results. Because symptom resolution seems to occur in no more than 20% to 30% of these patients after anti-*H. pylori* treatment and because of the complications associated with antibiotic use (e.g., reflux esophagitis), such therapy should not be recommended for this patient group.

REFERENCES

1. **Health and Public Policy Committee.** Endoscopy in the evaluation of dyspepsia. *Ann Intern Med.* 1985;102:266–9.

2. **El-Omar E, Penman I, Ardil JES, McColl KEL.** A substantial proportion of nonulcer dyspepsia patients have the same abnormality of acid secretion as duodenal ulcer patients. *Gut.* 1195;36:534–8.

3. **Armstrong D.** *Helicobacter pylori* infection and dyspepsia. *Scand J Gastroenterol.* 1996;31(Suppl 215):38–47.

4. **Holtmann G, Goebell H, Holtmann M, Talley NJ.** Dyspepsia in healthy blood

donors: pattern of symptoms and association with *Helicobacter pylori*. *Dig Dis Sci.* 1994;39:1090–8.

5. **Schlemper RJ, van der Werf S, Vandenbroucke JP, et al.** Nonulcer dyspepsia in a Dutch working population and *Helicobacter pylori*. *Arch Intern Med.* 1995;155: 82–7.

6. **Bernersen B, Johnsen R, Bostad L, et al.** Is *Helicobacter pylori* the cause of dyspepsia? *BMJ.* 1992;304:1976–9.

7. **Agreus L, Engstrand L, Svardsudd K, et al.** *Helicobacter* seropositivity among Swedish adults with and without abdominal symptoms: a population-based epidemiological study. *Scand J Gastroenterol.* 1995;30:752.

8. **Katelaris PH, Tippett GHK, Norbu P, et al.** Dyspepsia, *Helicobacter pylori*, and peptic ulcer in a randomly selected population in India. *Gut.* 1992;33:1462–6.

9. **Al-Moagel MA, Evans DG, Abdulghani ME, et al.** Prevalence of *Helicobacter pylori* infection in Saudi Arabia and comparison of those with and without upper gastrointestinal symptoms. *Am J Gastroenterol.* 1990;85;94–8.

10. **Gilvarry J, Buckley MJ, Beattie S, et al.** Eradication of *Helicobacter pylori* affects symptoms in nonulcer dyspepsia. *Scand J Gastroenterol.* 1997;32:535–40.

11. **Qvist N, Rasmussen L, Axelsonn CK.** *Helicobacter pylori* associated gastritis and dyspepsia: the influence on migrating motor complexes. *Scand J Gasrtoenterol.* 1994;29:133–7.

12. **Caballero-Plasencia AM, Muros-Navarro MC, Martin-Ruiz JL, et al.** Dyspeptic symptoms and gastric emptying of solids in patients with functional dyspepsia. *Scand J Gastroenterol.* 1995;30:745–51.

13. **Testoni PA, Bagnolo F, Bolongna P, et al.** Higher prevalence of *Helicobacter pylori* infection in dyspeptic patients who do not have phase III of the migrating motor complex. *Scand J Gastroenterol.* 1996;31:1063–8.

14. **Chang CS, Chen GH, Kao CH, et al.** The effect of *Helicobacter pylori* infection on gastric emptying of digestible and indigestible solids in patients with nonulcer dyspepsia. *Am J Gastroenterol.* 1996;91:474–9.

15. **Tucci A, Corinaldesi R, Stanghellini V, et al.** *Helicobacter pylori* infection and gastric function in patients with chronic idiopathic dyspepsia. *Gastroenterology.* 1992;103:768–74.

16. **Bechi P, Dei R, Amorosi A, et al.** *Helicobacter pylori* and luminal gastric pH: relationships in nonulcer dyspepsia. *Dig Dis Sci.* 1992;37:378–84.

17. **Mearin F, de Ribot X, Balboa A, et al.** Does *Helicobacter pylori* infection increase gastric sensitivity in functional dyspepsia? *Gut.* 1995;37:47–51.

18. **Holtmann G, Talley NJ, Goebell H.** Association between *Helicobacter pylori*, duodenal mechanosensory threshholds, and small intestinal motility in chronic unexplained dyspepsia. *Dig Dis Sci.* 1996;41:1285–91.

19. **Sheu BS, Lin CY, Lin XZ, et al.** Long-term outcome of triple therapy in *Helicobacter pylori*-related nonulcer dyspepsia: a prospective controlled assessment. *Am J Gastroenterol.* 1996;91:441–7.

20. **Lazzaroni M, Bargiggia S, Sangelatti O, et al.** Eradication of *Helicobacter pylori* and long-term outcome of functional dyspepsia: a clinical endoscopic study. *Dig Dis Sci.* 1996;41:1589–94.

21. **Blum AL, Talley NJ, O'Morain C, et al.** Lack of effect of treating *Helicobacter pylori* infection in patients with nonulcer dyspepsia. *N Engl J Med.* 1998;339:1875–81.

22. **McColl K, Murray L, El-Omar E, et al.** Symptomatic benefit from eradicating *Helicobacter pylori* infection in patients with nonulcer dyspepsia. *N Engl J Med.* 1998;339:1869–74.

23. **Talley NJ, Janssens J, Lauresten K, et al.** Eradication of *Helicobacter pylori* in functional dyspepsia: randomised, double-blind, placebo-controlled trial with 12-months' follow-up. *BMJ.* 1999;318:833–7.

24. **Fendrick AM, Chernew ME, Hirth RA, Bloom BS.** Alternative management strategies for patients with suspected peptic ulcer disease. *Ann Intern Med.* 1995; 123:260–8.

25. **Ofman JJ, Etchason J, Fullerton S, et al.** Management strategies for *Helicobacter pylori* seropositive patients with dyspepsia: clinical and economic consequences. *Ann Intern Med.* 1997;126:280–91.

26. **Silverstein MD, Petterson T, Talley NJ.** Initial endoscopy or empirical therapy with or without testing for *Helicobacter pylori* for dyspepsia: a decision analysis. *Gastroenterology.* 1996;110:72–83.

27. **Bytzer P, Hansen JM, Schaffalitzky de Muckadell OB.** Empirical H_2-blocker therapy or prompt endoscopy in management of dyspepsia. *Lancet.* 1994;343: 811–6.

28. **Balboa A, Zarate N, Cucala M, Malagelada JR.** Placebo in functional dyspepsia: symptomatic, gastrointestinal mctor, and gastric sensorial responses. *Am J Gastroenterol.* 1999;94:116–25.

29. **The European *Helicobacter* Study Group.** Current European concepts in the management of *Helicobacter pylori* infection. *Gut.* 1997;41:8–13.

5

Motility and Dyspepsia

Eammon M.M. Quigley, MD

A significant proportion of dyspepsia patients are not found to have underlying pathology, despite extensive investigation (1–3). By convention, this group is referred to as having functional (or "nonulcer") dyspepsia, and the pathophysiology, evaluation, and management of this group has been the focus of considerable emphasis in recent years (1). In any discussion of dyspepsia, it is important to be absolutely clear about what population of dyspepsia patients is under consideration, i.e., whether it is the entire population or solely those regarded as having functional dyspepsia. The term *functional* implies that organic causes of dyspepsia have been sought and eliminated. In developing evaluation and management strategies and algorithms in dyspepsia, another category has recently been referenced—the so-called *uninvestigated* dyspepsia. Although this group may well be dominated by those with functional dyspepsia, it does include many patients with dyspepsia of organic origin. These categories must not be confused.

Before discussing the evaluation and management of dysmotility in general, this review addresses two issues: 1) the contribution of primary disorders of gastrointestinal motor function to dyspepsia, and 2) the role of dysmotility in the pathophysiology of functional dyspepsia. It must be conceded from the outset that there is considerable blurring of the margins between these two issues—specifically the unresolved question of how one truly separates between "idiopathic" gastroparesis and gastroparesis documented in patients presenting with functional dyspepsia.

Dyspepsia as a Manifestation of the Primary Disorders of Gastrointestinal Motor Dysfunction

Although the most classic and characteristic symptom of gastroparesis is delayed postprandial vomiting of undigested food, many patients with established and severe gastrointestinal motor dysfunction that results in gastroparesis also exhibit dyspeptic-type symptoms. The various disease states that may be associated with gastroparesis are listed in Table 5.1. Indeed, any acute or chronic disorder that results in a diffuse disruption of gastrointestinal motor function may feature gastroparesis. Patients with established dysmotility, such as those with diabetic gastroparesis or chronic intestinal pseudo-obstruction, typically have severe disabling nausea and vomiting, resulting in weight loss and malnutrition. Among these patients, confusion with functional dyspepsia is unlikely. Although the diagnosis of gastroparesis is usually self-evident, its management is often challenging (4,5).

Table 5.1   Disease States That May Be Associated with Gastroparesis

Endocrine and Metabolic Diseases	*Surgical Outcomes*
• Diabetes mellitus	• Vagotomy
• Hypothyroidism	• Roux-en-Y syndrome
• Uremia	*Mucosal Diseases*
• Pregnancy	• Gastroesophageal reflux disease
• Amyloidosis	• Gastric ulceration
	• Viral gastritis
Neurological Diseases	
• Muscular dystrophy	*Other*
• Spinal cord disease	• Radiation therapy
• Parkinson's disease	• Anorexia nervosa
• Brain stem tumors	• Chronic liver disease
• Peripheral neuropathy	• Chronic intestinal pseudo-obstruction (primary and secondary)
Collagen Vascular Diseases	
• Scleroderma	
• Systemic lupus erythematosus	

Dysmotility in Functional Dyspepsia

For the purposes of this discussion, it must be emphasized that I am dealing with the patient who presents with functional dyspepsia and no other symptoms or signs suggestive of a primary or diffuse motor disorder as described in the preceding section. Unfortunately, the development of the concept of idiopathic gastroparesis has led to some confusion in this area (6). Until the basic pathophysiology of these instances of gastric motor dysfunction is understood and the precise role of gastric dysmotility in the pathogenesis of functional dyspepsia in general is clarified, confusion will continue. In the meantime, and for the purposes of this discussion, I have arbitrarily attempted to distinguish between 1) patients with clinically "obvious" manifestations of gastroparesis in whom no underlying cause can be identified (idiopathic gastroparesis), and 2) patients who present with dyspepsia and are found on investigation to have delayed gastric emptying.

The first (idiopathic gastroparesis) group presents with the classic gastroparesis symptoms (i.e., prominent vomiting [especially late postprandial], nausea, anorexia, and weight loss). Investigations suggest that gastric emptying delay and severe delay are confirmed on gastric emptying testing. In the second group, the presentation is indistinguishable from that of dyspepsia in general (i.e., predominant pain or discomfort centered in the upper abdomen) (1–3). In this group, symptomatology also may include early satiety, postprandial fullness, and nausea. Vomiting (which may be present but is not a prominent feature) and weight loss are usually not an issue. In these individuals, the initial clinical suspicion would not be delayed gastric emptying but rather gastric mucosal disease or peptic ulceration.

I acknowledge that future investigations may reveal that such a separation is completely without foundation and that these two conditions may represent the opposite ends of a single disease's spectrum. Pending such a resolution, however, I feel that a failure to describe this distinction will lead to an assumption that all dyspepsia is related to gastroparesis and that all patients presenting with even the vaguest complaint of upper abdominal discomfort should be subjected to tests of gastric motor function. Having established these ground rules and discussed some caveats, I examine the current status of gastric motor dysfunction in the pathogenesis of functional dyspepsia.

Definition of Gastric Dysmotility

Although motility has been regarded, for some time, as one of the most popular of several hypotheses advanced to explain the cause of functional dyspepsia, the interpretation of studies describing dysmotility in this patient population is fraught with problems. These problems begin with the very definition of the disorder (1,3). Given that this is a syndrome whose definition is entirely clinical, the inclusion or exclusion of certain symptoms may significantly bias the prevalence of dysmotility. For example, the inclusion of subjects with predominant bloating, early satiety, and vomiting may increase the proportion of patients who exhibit delayed gastric emptying or other features of gastric dysmotility. Similarly, the inclusion of patients with prominent heartburn also may increase the prevalence of gastroparesis, given the reported association between gastroesophageal reflux disease and delayed gastric emptying (5). Currently, a more restricted definition of dyspepsia holds sway, emphasizing the predominance of pain or discomfort in the upper abdomen and excluding those who have predominant reflux (1). Given the known overlap between dyspepsia and reflux, the separation of these disorders may be achieved more readily in theory than in practice (3,7,8). Overlap with other functional disorders (irritable bowel syndrome in particular) also influences the prevalence of other motor and sensory phenomena in a given patient population (9). Furthermore, the location of a study influences its outcome; thus, studies of patients with "resistant" dyspepsia who are investigated in tertiary referral centers are likely to yield a significantly different perspective on the pathophysiology of functional dyspepsia than those performed in the community (10).

Role of Gastrointestinal Motor Dysfunction in the Pathogenesis of Functional Dyspepsia

Of the various parameters of motor function that have been studied in these patients, gastric emptying has achieved the most attention. In a variety of studies, delayed gastric emptying has been demonstrated in 25% to 40% of patients with functional dyspepsia (11–20). The interpretation of this finding is controversial, and the relationships between gastroparesis, symptoms, prognosis, and therapeutic response remain unclear. Other studies using electrogastrography have identified a similar prevalence of gastric electrical dysrhythmias (18,21–24). The relationship of these findings to symptoms and gastric motor function also remains unclear, and a role has yet to be established for this relatively noninvasive technology in the assessment of dyspepsia (25–28).

Relationships Between Gastric Emptying Rate and Symptoms

Recently, Stanghellini and coworkers (16) studied the predictive value of symptoms that are suggestive of gastroparesis in 343 patients with functional dyspepsia. Forty percent of their female patients proved to have gastroparesis; however, the average degree of gastric emptying delay was only approximately 30% above normal. Even among this selected group, it was difficult to predict a motor abnormality on the basis of symptoms. When the authors evaluated whether the presence or absence of a particular symptom could predict gastroparesis, they found that postprandial fullness alone was predictive. On multiple regression analysis, female gender alone predicted gastroparesis and, when symptoms were evaluated according to severity, relevant and severe (or "predominant") postprandial fullness, nausea, and vomiting were more prevalent among those with delayed gastric emptying (16). Other studies have emphasized the value of other predominant symptoms in identifying pathophysiologic subgroups; thus, heartburn predicts both reflux (29) and a painful ulcer-type dyspepsia that is responsive to acid suppression (30).

Studies of prokinetic agents also have made the discrepancies between symptoms, gastric emptying rate, and therapeutic response abundantly clear. Although cisapride has been shown in both short- and long-term studies to accelerate gastric emptying, this does not necessarily predict a symptomatic response (31,32). Furthermore, in a recent multicenter study in the United States, domperidone produced a modest improvement in symptoms among patients with diabetic gastroenteropathy, regardless of gastric emptying results (33,34). I would suggest, therefore, that the true significance of a modest delay in gastric emptying in dyspepsia patients has not been resolved. This is important because there has been a rush to ascribe symptoms to a scintigraphic study result, although this may be no more than a mere epiphenomenon. A preoccupation with "gastroparesis" in this situation may lead to a failure to identify the true primary pathology and, accordingly, to initiate or delay appropriate therapy.

Abnormalities Associated with Pathogenesis of Functional Dyspepsia

Given the recognition of distinct functions within various regions of the stomach, several authors recently have evaluated the function of these physiologically distinct parts of the stomach in dyspepsia patients. Manometric studies have identified antral postprandial hypomotility as a relatively common abnormality among patients with functional dyspepsia, especially among those with gastroparesis (11–13,35–39). Again, for reasons that are unclear, this abnormality is more common among women; however, this finding is notoriously nonspecific. It also has been documented among patients with peptic ulcer disease, diabetic gastroparesis, and intestinal pseudo-obstruction and can be induced in normal subjects on exposure to an appropriate stress (5). The significance of the abnormal duodenal motor patterns reported in a few studies is similarly unclear (35–41). Specifically, do these "abnormalities" signify a primary abnormality of the gastrointestinal motor apparatus, or are they also mere epiphenomena secondary to an as-yet-unidentified primary pathology (as in the case of gastroparesis)?

Evidence for regional gastric dysfunction in dyspepsia was first demonstrated in detailed gastric emptying studies preformed by Troncon and coworkers (42,43). Among a group of dyspeptics who demonstrated normal emptying of a solid meal, they noted abnormalities in intragastric distribution. The meal was emptied more rapidly from the proximal stomach; however, emptying from the distal stomach was delayed (42). Further studies have supported this finding (20,44–46). Thus, Tack and coworkers (20) found that approximately 40% of a relatively large group of patients with functional dyspepsia demonstrated impaired relaxation of the upper stomach. In other studies that addressed the function of the distal stomach, the antrum appeared more distended among subjects with functional dyspepsia in both fasting and postprandial states (47–51). This finding is of particular interest because studies in normal volunteers have demonstrated a close relationship between the development of postprandial fullness and the extent of antral expansion (52). Similarly, early satiety and bloating seem to have an inverse correlation with postprandial fundic volume (20,53).

These various studies suggest, with reasonable consistency, that subtle and dynamic changes in regional volume or distension of the stomach may have an important role to play in the genesis of dyspeptic symptoms (25). It is tempting, although perhaps premature, to integrate these various findings into the unifying hypothesis that follows. In this scenario, a failure of the proximal stomach to relax adequately on meal ingestion leads to premature diversion of the meal to the antrum, which in turn causes antral distention and symptom provocation. On manometric studies, antral dilation by itself results in apparent antral hypomotility. More extreme and sustained degrees of distension could, of course, lead to actual impairment of antral contractile force and, thus, to a delay in emptying of solid particles from the stomach (i.e., gastroparesis). This proposal does not assume that abnormal fundic relaxation is the primary phenomenon. What it *does* attempt to do is bring a number of strands of evidence derived from disparate studies of gastric motor activity into a unifying concept.

Role of Other Mechanisms in the Pathogenesis of Functional Dyspepsia

Motility is not, of course, the only proposed pathophysiology of functional dyspepsia. Indeed, dysmotility may interact with a number of these other proposed mechanisms. Although there is little evidence for a direct effect of *Helicobacter pylori* infection on such motor parameters as gastric emptying, antral motility, or fundic relaxation (15,19,54-58), this organism may interact with other factors to promote gastric hypersensitivity (26). Given the demonstrated effects of cytokines and other inflammatory mediators on gut muscle and nerve function, it does not seem unreasonable to expect that the chronic inflammation induced by *H. pylori* infection could alter foregut motor physiology. However, the role of *H. pylori* in the pathogenesis of symptoms in nonulcer dyspepsia remains controversial at best (19).

In contrast, the concept of visceral hypersensitivity has gained increasing currency. Carefully controlled studies have demonstrated a lower threshold of gastric and intestinal distension in patients with functional dyspepsia (24,43,46,59–62). The anatomic sites of this abnormal sensitivity are unknown. Several possibilities exist, including up-regulation of sensory receptors in the gut wall, abnormal activation of afferent neurons, and heightened perception within the central nervous system (CNS). CNS dysfunction, of course, also could modulate peripheral sensation by enhancing gastric tone or phasic motor activity. In this manner, motor and sensory phenomena could be influenced even by psychological factors. Evidence does exist for central dysfunction in dyspepsia, including both abnormalities in the central neuroendocrine axis (63) and disturbances in sleep and nocturnal gastrointestinal motor patterns (40). Although delineating the primacy of one of these factors in the etiology of symptoms will continue to pose a daunting challenge, the importance of disentangling this pathophysiologic web is obvious, given the potential availability of specific agonists and antagonists to a variety of receptors at various levels of control within the central, autonomic, and enteric nervous systems.

Recent studies also have emphasized the limitations and potential pitfalls of studying proposed pathophysiologic mechanisms in isolation (64). For example, it is increasingly evident that dysmotility and sensation may not operate in isolation but may be intimately related. Meal-related symptoms in dyspepsia patients may well be based more on interactions between gastric tone and distention than on primary motor events and resultant changes in gastric emptying rate. Thus, altered gastric tone (a motor event) clearly resets the threshold for sensitivity to distention (65). Interactions between parts of the gut also may play a role. In dyspepsia, impaired gastric accommodation may be the consequence of gastric hyporesponsiveness to the duodenogastric reflex that normally promotes fundic relaxation when the duodenum is distended (61). This impaired accommodation response to meal ingestion or duodenal stimulation exaggerates any pre-existing hypersensitivity to distension within the proximal stomach, thereby accentuating postprandial symptoms. Experimental studies also have shown that afferent input can directly modulate motility through reflexes intrinsic to the gut wall and mediated through the enteric nervous system or the autonomic and central nervous systems. For these reasons, it is also not unreasonable to speculate that some of the abnormal patterns documented in dyspepsia may not be primary phenomena but rather may represent a motor response to afferent sensory traffic.

In summary, although the dyspepsia field has generated several interesting and potentially important hypotheses, the primacy of any one of these phenomena remains to be established. It is possible that future research may identify subgroups of patients in whom a particular pathophysiologic phenomenon predominates. Alternatively, as suggested by studies indicating interactions between the CNS, gastric motor activity, and gastric sensation, these phenomena may interact to reinforce or enhance symptoms. It also remains distinctly possible that all of these may be mere epiphenomena generated by another yet-to-be-identified primary abnormality.

The Evaluation of Gastrointestinal Motor Function

Before considering motor dysfunction, and being mindful of the nonspecificity of dyspepsia symptoms (3), the clinician should ensure that mucosal or mechanical causes have been ruled out. In particular, give consideration to peptic ulcer disease, gastroesophageal reflux disease, and low-grade intestinal obstruction. Review medications carefully to identify iatrogenic causes of nausea and vomiting, and keep in mind the possible contribution of psychological factors (depression in particular).

If, at this stage, symptoms remain unexplained and underlying dysmotility is suspected, two options are available. One begins with a screening test of gastric function, such as gastric emptying scintigraphy (or electrogastrography), and further therapy is based on its result. The second approach is to initiate empirical therapy with a prokinetic or prokinetic/anti-emetic combination. Testing in this approach is limited to patients who do not respond to therapy. In either strategy, more detailed and invasive tests of motor function, such as manometry, are reserved for those with persistent and disabling symptoms who do not respond satisfactorily to empirical therapy.

For decades, scintigraphy has been the most widely performed test for gastric emptying (5). Although this may be performed using either solid or liquid markers, solid-phase markers (e.g., chicken liver, scrambled eggs) have been the most widely employed and validated. It is important to bear in mind that gastric emptying rates are influenced by several technical factors that may vary considerably between centers. For this reason, it is recommended that each laboratory develop its own normal values. Recently, a simplified protocol has been shown to provide reproducible results with acceptable variability among centers in a multicenter study (66). Scintigraphy does involve radiation exposure and requires considerable gamma-camera time. For this reason, the recent introduction of a gastric emptying test based on the excretion of the stable isotope ^{14}C in the breath has been greeted with considerable enthusiasm. The subject ingests ^{14}C-octanoic acid, and breath sampling is performed for 6 hours. Initial studies suggest that this may be an acceptable test of gastric emptying, which could be performed in the doctor's office (67,68). An abnormal scintigraphy is reported when the $T_{1/2}$ emptying time is delayed compared with that of normal subjects.

Electrogastrography (EGG) has been advocated as a screening test of gastric dysmotility (21,22,69). It is performed by placing electrodes (similar to those used for electrocardiography) over the surface markings of the stomach. Although results of EGG studies have been shown, in general, to parallel those of gastric emptying tests, they are by no means equivalent (21) and, until further data are available, one cannot recommend the EGG as a substitute for gastric emptying scintigraphy for evaluating gastric motor function (28). The EGG may provide insights into physiology and pathophysiology, which may be important; however, at this time, the clinical relevance of this information remains unclear. Other approaches to the assessment of gastric motor function (e.g., magnetic resonance imaging, ultrasound, impedance) remain within the realm of clinical research (26).

Management of Dysmotility in Dyspepsia Patients

When managing the patient with functional dyspepsia and gastrointestinal dysmotility, several factors need to be addressed (5). A discussion of nutritional issues and pharmacologic management follows.

Nutritional Status

Attention to nutritional status is of paramount importance. Specific deficiencies should be identified and appropriate replacement instituted. In patients with gastroparesis, a low-fat, low-residue diet should be instituted, given the known effects of these dietary factors on gastric emptying rate (and on bezoar formation in diabetes patients). Initially, every attempt should be made to institute an adequate nutritional intake via the oral route by using diets of variable composition and consistency and by adding appropriate oral supplements. However, for the gastroparesis patient who cannot tolerate or achieve an adequate caloric intake by the oral route either in the short or long term, a number of alternatives are available. Short-term enteral nutrition can be delivered via nasogastric or nasoenteric tube. If long-term oral intake cannot be reinstituted, access to the gastrointestinal tract may be achieved through a gastrostomy or jejunostomy. One approach is to commence enteral feeding via the nasogastric or nasoenteric route on a trial basis; if this is tolerated, a jejunostomy can be performed for long-term nutrition intake. In patients with severe gastroparesis, gastrostomy feeding by definition may prove unsuccessful; however, it may help by allowing the patient to periodically "vent" the stomach and relieve distressing distension and bloating. Indeed, one approach to the management of patients with severe intractable gastroparesis is the simultaneous placement of a gastrostomy for venting and a jejunostomy for enteral feeding.

Pharmacologic Therapy

Prokinetics and anti-emetics are the primary pharmacologic agents available for the management of patients with symptomatic gastroparesis and dyspepsia in general (Table 5.2). The first prokinetic agents were nonspecific cholinergic agonists, such as bethanechol. Although these agents are capable of stimulating gastric emptying (70), there is little evidence for efficacy in gastrointestinal motor disorders, and their use was complicated by a high

Table 5.2   Drugs Used in the Pharmacologic Treatment of Dyspepsia-Associated Gastroparesis

Drug	Recommended Dosage	Advantages	Disadvantages	Comments
Prokinetic agents				
Metoclopramide	10–15 mg every half-hour AC + qhs (oral or IV)	Used for the short-term symptomatic treatment of diabetic gastroparesis; available in several formulations; has anti-emetic properties	CNS- and hyperpro-lactinemia-related side effects with long-term use; tachyphylaxis (tolerance benefit)	Can be given sub-cutaneously in patients who do not respond to an oral regimen
Domperidone	10–20 mg every half-hour AC + qhs	Symptomatic treat-ment of diabetic gastroparesis; no extrapyramidal side effects (e.g., those experienced with metoclopra-mide); has anti-emetic properties	Risk of hyper-prolactinemia; not available in U.S.	
Cisapride	10–20 mg every half-hour AC + qhs (oral)	Accelerates liquid and solid empty-ing over short and long terms	Has potential to induce cardiac conduction and rhythm disturbance*	Removed from U.S. market; available on a restricted basis[†]
Erythromycin	50–250 mg every 6 hours (oral or IV)	Corrects gastro-paresis even in refractory patients who require hospitalization	Long-term dosing problems in outpatients	
Anti-emetic agents[‡]				
Prochlorperazine	0.15–0.45 mg/kg every 4–8 hours	Effective and inex-pensive (generic)	Hypertension, drowsiness, extrapyramidal side effects	Not for use in children
Ondansetron	0.15–0.45 mg/kg every 4–8 hours	Extremely effective 5HT-3 agonist; works at enteric nervous system and chemo-receptor for trigger zone	Headache, broncho-spasm, tachy-cardia; expensive	Available in an oral formulation

AC = before meals; CNS = central nervous system; IV = intravenous.

* Because of these cardiac disturbances, cisapride is contraindicated in patients who take agents that are known to inhibit cytochrome P450 3A4 metabolism or in those predisposed to cardiac conduction or rhythm abnormalities.

[†] Cisapride is available only for individual use in a highly select group of patients. Contact Jannsen Pharmaceutica for an application.

[‡] Metoclopramide and domperidone also have anti-emetic actions (see separate entries above).

prevalence of side effects outside of the gastrointestinal tract. Therefore, metoclopramide (a dopamine antagonist) represented a significant advance in prokinetic therapy (70). Through its central actions, metoclopramide is an effective anti-emetic—its peripheral actions lead to an acceleration of gastric emptying and promote esophageal motor activity. Although metoclopramide has been shown to be effective in the short term, its long-term use in the symptomatic therapy of diabetic gastroparesis has been complicated by tolerance issues and a relatively high prevalence of CNS- and hyperprolactinemia-related side effects. However, one advantage of metoclopramide is its availability in different formulations, such as for oral (both tablet and suspension forms) and subcutaneous administration. Domperidone (another dopamine antagonist) does not cross the blood-brain barrier and, therefore, is not associated with the extrapyramidal side effects that have complicated metoclopramide use. Domperidone is both anti-emetic and prokinetic, and it has been shown to be valuable in the symptomatic management of patients with diabetic gastroparesis (71) and of diabetes patients with dyspepsia symptoms in general (33,34). However, it may cause hyperprolactinemia.

Cisapride (available in tablet and suspension forms) facilitates acetylcholine release in the enteric nervous system through a 5HT-4–mediated effect and has been shown to promote motor activity along the length of the gastrointestinal tract (see Table 5.2). It also has been shown to accelerate liquid and solid emptying in both the short (6 weeks) (31) and long (>1 year) (32) terms. Thus, it has become an important component of the management of patients with gastroparesis and other gastrointestinal motor disorders. Recently, however, concerns have been raised about its potential to induce cardiac conduction and rhythm disturbances, especially when employed in conjunction with agents that either modify its metabolism or are prone to prolong the Q-T interval. Cisapride should not be used in conjunction with agents known to inhibit cytochrome P450 3A4 metabolism in the liver or in individuals predisposed to cardiac conduction or rhythm abnormalities (72).

Erythromycin acts as a motilin agonist to stimulate motor activity, primarily in the upper gastrointestinal tract (73) (see Table 5.2). When given intravenously, low-dose erythromycin (50–100 mg) is a potent gastroprokinetic agent and corrects gastroparesis effectively, even in patients with refractory symptoms. Thus, intravenous erythromycin has become an important component of the management of patients with intractable gastroparesis, particularly those who require hospitalization. Oral erythromycin has proven disappointing, even when used in suspension form (74). Whether this reflects the relatively poor bioavailability of this agent or the development of tolerance remains unclear. The latter seems less likely given the recent demonstration of its long-term (up to 18 months) efficacy when given intravenously to patients with refractory gastroparesis (75). Given that this is an antibiotic and also a potent inhibitor of the hepatic cytochrome system, this approach should be regarded as a last resort in patients with the most intractable symptoms. Several related compounds are currently under investigation, with the goal being to produce an agent with prokinetic properties similar to that of erythromycin but effective when administered orally and devoid of antibiotic activity.

Nausea is a prominent symptom in patients with diabetic and idiopathic gastropathy. Many of these patients find awakening each morning with nausea a more distressing symptom than vomiting. For this reason, anti-emetic agents assume an important therapeutic role. Some prokinetic agents (metoclopramide and domperidone) have anti-emetic actions, whereas others (cisapride and erythromycin) do not. Therefore, in patients with nausea, an anti-emetic (e.g., a phenothiazine derivative or a 5HT-3 antagonist) should be used in conjunction with a prokinetic agent; often these drugs can be taken successfully on an as-needed basis. When choosing a particular anti-emetic, pay attention to the appropriateness of available formulations, duration of action, and cost.

Recently, gastric pacing has been proposed as an alternative for those with intractable gastroparesis (76,77). Although the precise mode of action of gastric stimulation remains uncertain (78)—and may be independent of an acceleration of gastric emptying—the results of two pilot studies were impressive enough to warrant further study.

Prokinetic agents have been used widely and studied among patients with functional dyspepsia. Their use has been based on the assumption that dysmotility is a factor in the pathogenesis of this disorder. Recent meta-analyses have suggested that these agents (domperidone and cisapride in particular) have modest efficacy in dyspepsia (79,80), but attempts to relate this response to a correction of motor dysfunction have not been convincing (33,81). Indeed, the question of whether their use should be restricted to those with dysmotility remains unresolved; several other factors, such as a central anti-emetic effect in the case of domperidone or a modulation of gastric tone or visceral sensation (59,82), could explain their ability to resolve symptoms in some patients.

Conclusions

Dysmotility may contribute to the development of dyspeptic symptoms either through the gross perturbations of motor function characteristics of the patient with severe gastroparesis or through the more subtle and, perhaps, regional disturbances of motility described in patients with functional dyspepsia in general. We have much more to learn about the relationships among symptoms, disturbed physiology, and therapeutic response (83).

Recommendations

- When the cause of dyspepsia is suspected to be dysmotility, diagnostic evaluation should begin either with a screening test of gastric motor function (e.g., gastric emptying scintigraphy, electrogastrography) or with empirical therapy of prokinetics or a prokinetic/anti-emetic combination.

- For patients with persistent and disabling symptoms and those who do not respond satisfactorily to empirical therapy, more detailed and invasive tests of motor function (e.g., manometry) may be considered.

- Management involves ensuring adequate nutritional assessment and support and pharmacologic therapy as outlined in this chapter.

- Endoscopic or surgical approaches should be considered when the aforementioned methods fail.

Key Points

- In many patients with gastrointestinal motor dysfunction, dyspepsia may be an early manifestation of the disorder.

- The significance of a modest delay in gastric emptying in dyspepsia patients has not been resolved.

- Antral postprandial hypomotility has been linked to the pathogenesis of functional dyspepsia.

- In the pathogenesis of functional dyspepsia, dysmotility may interact with other mechanisms, such as visceral hypersensitivity, altered gastric tone, and afferent input.

- Further research is needed to identify a predominant pathophysiologic phenomenon.

- Evaluation for gastrointestinal dysmotility may begin with a screening test, such as scintigraphy, or with empirical therapy using prokinetic agents.

- Management of gastrointestinal dysmotility includes ensuring adequate nutritional intake and pharmacologic therapy to correct gastroparesis and dysfunction in motor activity and to suppress symptoms such as nausea. Endoscopic or surgical approaches also may need to be considered.

REFERENCES

1. **Talley NJ, Silverstein MD, Agreus L, et al.** AGA technical review: evaluation of dyspepsia. *Gastroenterology.* 1998;114:582–95.

2. **Talley NJ, Colin-Jones D, Koch KJ, et al.** Functional dyspepsia: a classification with guidelines for diagnosis and management. *Gastroenterol Int.* 1991;4:145–60.

3. **Crean GP, Holden RJ, Knill-Jones RP, et al.** A database on dyspepsia. *Gut.* 1994; 35:191–202.

4. **Quigley EMM.** Intestinal pseudo-obstruction. In Champion MC, Orr WC (eds). *Evolving Concepts in Gastrointestinal Motil.* Oxford, England: Blackwell Science; 1996:171–99.

5. **Quigley EMM.** Gastic and small intestinal motility in health and disease. *Gastroenterol Clin North Am.* 1996;25:113–145.

6. **Soykan I, Sivri B, Sarosiek I, et al.** Demography, clinical characteristics, psychological and abuse profiles, treatment, and long-term follow-up of patients with gastroparesis. *Dig Dis Sci.* 1998;43:2398–404.

7. **Talley NJ, Zinsmeister AR, Schleck CD, Melton LJ III.** Dyspepsia and dyspepsia subgroups: population-based study. *Gastroenterology.* 1992;102:1259–68.

8. **Small PK, Loudon MA, Waldron B, et al.** Importance of reflux symptoms in functional dyspepsia. *Gut.* 1995;36:189–92.

9. **Agreus L, Svardsudd K, Nyren O, Tibblin G.** Irritable bowel syndrome and dyspepsia in the general population: overlap and lack of stability over time. *Gasteroenterology.* 1995;109:671–80.

10. **Whitehead WE, Winget C, Fedoravicius AS, et al.** Learned illness behaviour in patients with irritable bowel syndrome and peptic ulcer disease. *Dig Dis Sci.* 1982; 27:702–8.

11. **Labo G, Bortolotti M, Vezzadini P, et al.** Interdigestive gastroduodenal motility and serum motilin levels in patients with idiopathic delay in gastric emptying. *Gastroenterology.* 1986;90:20–6.

12. **Kerlin P.** Postprandial antral hypomotility in patients with idiopathic nausea and vomiting. *Gut.* 1989;30:54–9.

13. **Waldron B, Cullen PT, Kumar R, et al.** Evidence for hypomotility in nonulcer dyspepsia: a prospective multifactorial study. *Gut.* 1991;32:246–51.

14. **Jian R, Ducrot F, Ruskone A, et al.** Symptomatic, radionuclide, and therapeutic assessement of chronic idiopathic dyspepsia: a double-blind placebo-controlled evaluation of dyspepsia. *Dig Dis Sci.* 1989;34:657–64.

15. **Scott AM, Kellow JE, Shuter B, et al.** Intragastric distribution and gastric emptying of solids and liquids in functional dyspepsia: lack of influence of symptom subgroups and *Helicobacter pylori* infection. *Dig Dis Sci.* 1993;38:2247–54.

16. **Stanghellini V, Toetti C, Patermico A, et al.** Risk indicators of delayed gastric emptying of solids in patients with functional dyspepsia. *Gastroenterology.* 1996; 110:1036–42.

17. **Maes BD, Ghoos YF, Hiele MI, Rutgeerts PJ.** Gastric emptying rate of solids in patients with nonulcer dyspepsia. *Dig Dis Sci.* 1997;42:1158–62.

18. **Pfaffenbach B, Adamek RJ, Bartholomans C, Wegener M.** Gastric dysrhythmias and delayed gastric emptying in patients with functional dyspepsia. *Dig Dis Sci.* 1997;42:2094–9.

19. **Fock KM, Khoo TK, Chia KS, Sing CS.** *Helicobacter pylori* infection and gastric emptying of indigestible solids in patients with dysmotility-like dyspepsia. *Scand J.Gastroenterol.* 1997;32:676–80.

20. **Tack J, Piessevuax H, Coulie B, et al.** Role of impaired gastric accommodation to a meal in functional dyspepsia. *Gastroenterology.* 1998;115:1346–52.

21. **Chen JDZ, Lin ZY, Pan J, McCallum RW.** Abnormal gastric myoelectrical activity and delayed gastric emptying in patients with symptoms suggestive of gastroparesis. *Dig Dis Sci.* 1996;41:1538–45.

22. **Parkman HP, Miller MA, Trate D, et al.** Electrogastrography and gastric emptying scintigraphy are complementary for assessment of dyspepsia. *J Clin Gastro.* 1997;24:214–9.

23. **Geldof H, Van Der Schee EJ, Van Blankenstein M, Grashuis JL.** Electrogastrographic study of gastric myoelectrical activity in patients with unexplained nausea and vomiting. *Gut.* 1986;27:799–808.

24. **Koch Kl, Medina M, Bingaman S, et al.** Gastric dysrhythmias and visceral sensation in patients with functional dyspepsia. *Gasteroenterolgy.* 1991;101:999–1006.

25. **Quigley EMM.** Symptoms and gastric function in dyspepsia: goodbye to gastroparesis? *Neurogastroenteroi and Motil.* 1996;8:273–6.

26. **Quigley EMM.** Gastroduodenal motility. *Curr Opin Gastroenterol.* 1997;13:479–84.

27. **Quigley EMM.** Gastroduodenal motility. *Curr Opin Gastroenterol.* 1998;14:437–446.

28. **Camilleri M, Hasher WL, Parkman HP, et al.** Measurement of gastrointestinal motility in the GI laboratory. *Gastroenterology.* 1998;115:747–62.

29. **Klauser AG, Schindlbeck NE, Muller-Lissner SA.** Symptoms in gastro-oesophageal reflux disease. *Lancet.* 1990;335:205–8.

30. **Talley NJ, Meineche-Schmidt V, Pare P, et al.** Efficacy of omeprazole in functional dyspepsia: double-blind, randomized, placebo-controlled trials (the Bond and Opera studies). *Aliment Pharmacol Ther.* 1998;12:1055–65.

31. **Camilleri M, Malagelada JR, Abell TL, et al.** Effect of six weeks of treatment with cisapride in gastroparesis and intestinal pseudo-obstruction. *Gastroenterology.* 1989;96:704–12.

32. **Abell TL, Camilleri M, DiMagno EP, et al.** Long-term efficacy of oral cisapride in symptomatic upper gut dysmotility. *Dig Dis Sci.* 1991;36:616–20.

33. **Silvers D, Kipnes M, Broadstone V, the DOM-USA-5 study group.** Domperidone in the management of symptoms of diabetic gastroparesis: efficacy, safety and quality-of-life outcomes in a multicenter controlled trial. *Clin Ther.* 1998;20:438–53.

34. **Farup CE, Leidy NY, Murray M, et al.** Effect of domperidone on the health-related quality of life of patients with symptoms of diabetic gastroparesis. *Diabetes Care.* 1998;21:1699–1706.

35. **Malagelada J-R, Stanghellini V.** Manometric evaluation of functional upper gut symptoms. *Gastroenterology.* 1985;88:1223–31.

36. **Bassotti G, Pelli MA, Morelli A.** Duodenojejunal motor activity in patients with chronic dyspeptic symptoms. *J Clin Gastroenterol.* 1990:12:17–21.

37. **Stanghellini V, Ghidini C, Maccarini MR, et al.** Fasting and postprandial gastrointestinal motility in ulcer and nonulcer dyspepsia. *Gut.* 1992;33:184–90.

38. **Jebbink HJA, Van Berge-Henegouwen GP, Akkermans LMA, et al.** Antroduodenal manometry: 24-hour ambulatory monitoring versus short-term stationary manometry in patients with functional dyspepsia. *Eur J Gastroenterol Hepatol.* 1995;7:109–16.

39. **Jebbink HJA, Van Berge-Henegouwen GP, Akkermans LMA, et al.** Small intestinal motor abnormalities in patients with functional dyspepsia demonstrated by ambulatory manometry. *Gut.* 1996;38:694–700.

40. **David D, Mertz H, Fefer L, et al.** Sleep and duodenal motor activity in patients with severe non-ulcer dyspepsia. *Gut.* 1994;35:916–25.

41. **Wilmer A, Van Cutsem E, Andrioli A, et al.** Prolonged ambulatory gastrojejunal manometry in severe motility-like dyspepsia: lack of correlation between dysmotility symptoms and gastric emptying. *Gut.* 1998;42:36–41.

42. **Troncon LEA, Bennett RJM, Ahluwahlia NK, Thompson DG.** Abnormal distribution of food during gastric emptying in functional dyspepsia patients. *Gut.* 1994; 35:327–32.

43. **Troncon LEA, Thompson DG, Ahluwahlia NK, et al.** Relations between upper abdominal symptoms and gastric distension abnormalities in dysmotility-like functional dyspepsia and after vagotomy. *Gut.* 1995;37:17–22.

44. **Gilja OH, Detmer PR, Jong JM, et al.** Intragastric distribution and gastric emptying assessed by three-dimensional ultrasonography. *Gastroenterology.* 1997;113: 38–49.

45. **Gilja OH, Hausken T, Wilhelmsen I, Berstad A.** Impaired accommodation of proximal stomach to a meal in functional dyspepsia. *Dig Dis Sci.* 1996;41:689–96.

46. **Salet GAM, Samsom A, Roelofs JMM, et al.** Responses to gastric distension in functional dyspepsia. *Gut.* 1998;42:823–9.

47. **Hausken T, Berstad A.** Wide gastric antrum in patients with nonulcer dyspepsia: effect of cisapride. *Scand. J Gastroenterol.* 1992;27:427–32.

48. **Ricci R, Bontempo I, LaBella A, et al.** Dyspeptic symptoms and gastric antrum distribution: an ultrasonographic study. *Ital J Gastroenterol.* 1987;19:215–7.

49. **Undeland KA, Hausken T, Svebak S, et al.** Wide gastric antrum and low vagal tone in patients with diabetes mellitus type 1 compared to patients with functional dyspepsia and healthy individuals. *Dig Dis Sci.* 1996;41:9–16.

50. **Ahluwahlia NK, Thompson DG, Mamtora H, et al.** Evaluation of gastric antral motor performance in patients with dysmotility-like dyspepsia using real-time high resolution ultrasound. *Neurogastroenterol Motil.* 1996;8:332–8.

51. **Hausken T, Thune N, Matre K, et al.** Volume estimation of the gastric antrum and the gall bladder in patients with nonulcer dyspepsia and erosive prepyloric changes, using three-dimensional ultrasonography. *Neurogastroenterol Motil.* 1994; 6:263–70.

52. **Jones KL, Doran SM, Hveem K, et al.** Relation between post-prandial satiation and antral area in normal subjects. *Am J Clin Nutr.* 1997;66:127–32.

53. **Samsom M, Roelofs JMM, Akkermans LMA, et al.** Proximal gastric motor activity in response to a liquid meal in type 1 diabetes mellitus with autonomic neuropathy. *Dig Dis Sci.* 1998;43:491–6.

54. **Tucci A, Corinaldesi R, Stanghellini V, et al.** *Helicobacter pylori* infection and gastric function in patients with chronic idiopathic dyspepsia. *Gastroenterology.* 1992;103:768–74.

55. **Pieramico O, Ditschuneit H, Malfertheiner P.** Gastrointestinal motility in patients with nonulcer dyspepsia: a role for *Helicobacter pylori* infection? *Am J Gastroenterol.* 1993;88:364–8.

56. **Mearin F, Ribot X, Balboa A, et al.** Does *Helicobacter pylori* infection increase gastric sensitivity in functional dyspepsia? *Gut.* 1995;37:47–51.

57. **Holtmann G, Talley NJ, Goebell H.** Association between *Helicobacter pylori*, duodenal mechanosensory thresholds, and small intestinal motility in chronic unexplained dyspepsia. *Dig Dis Sci.* 1996;41:1285–91.

58. **Saslow SB, Thumshirn M, Camilleri M, et al.** Influence of *Helicobacter pylori* infection on gastric motor and sensory function in asymptomatic volunteers. *Dig Dis Sci.* 1998;43:258–64.

59. **Bradette M, Pare P, Douville P, Morin A.** Visceral perception in health and functional dyspepsia: crossover study of gastric distensions with placebo and domperidone. *Dig Dis Sci.* 1991;36:52–8.

60. **Mearin F, Cucala M, Azpiroz F, Malagelada JR.** The origin of symptoms on the brain: gut axis in functional dyspepsia. *Gastroenterology.* 1991;101:996–1006.

61. **Coffin B, Azpiroz F, Guarner F, Malagelada JR.** Selective gastric hypersensitivity and reflex hyporeactivity in functional dyspepsia. *Gastroenterology.* 1994;107:1345–51.

62. **Lemann M, Dederding JP, Flourie, et al.** Abnormal perception of visceral pain in response to gastric distention in chronic idiopathic dyspepsia: the irritable stomach. *Dig Dis Sci.* 1991;36:1249–54.

63. **Chua A, Keating J, Hamilton D, et al.** Central serotonin receptors and delayed gastric emptying in nonulcer dyspepsia. *BMJ.* 1992;305:280–2.

64. **Moragas G, Azpiroz F, Pavia J, et al.** Relations among intragastric pressure, postcibal perception and gastric empyting. *Am J Physiol.* 1943;264:G1112–7.

65. **Notivol R, Coffin B, Azpiroz F, et al.** Gastric tone determines the sensitivity of the stomach to distension. *Gastroenterology.* 1995;108:330–6.

66. **Tougas G, McCallum RW, Abell TL, et al.** Simplified scintigraphic assessment of gastric emptying using a low fat meal: establishment of international control values. In press.

67. **Ghoos YF, Maes BD, Geypens BJ, et al.** Measurement of gastric emptying rate of solids by means of a carbon-labelled octanoic acid breath test. *Gastroenterology.* 1993;104:1640–7.

68. **Choi M-G, Camilleri M, Burton DD, et al.** 13C Octanoic acid breath test for gastric emptying of solids: accuracy, reproducibility and comparison with scintigraphy. *Gastroenterology.* 1997;112:1155–62.

69. **Chen JDZ, McCallum RW.** Clinical applications of electrogastrography. *Am J Gastroenterol.* 1993;88:1324–36.

70. **Malagelada JR, Rees WDW, Mazzotta J, Go VLW.** Gastric motor abnormalities in diabetic and postvagotomy gastroparesis: effect of metoclopramide and bethanechol. *Gastroenterology.* 1980;78:286–93.

71. **Horowitz M, Harding PE, Chatterton BE, et al.** Acute and chronic effects of domperidone on gastric emptying in diabetic autonomic neuropathy. *Dig Dis Sci.* 1985;30:1–9.

72. **Bedford TA, Rowbotham DJ.** Cisapride: drug interactions of clinical significance. *Drug Safety.* 1996;15:167–75.

73. **Camilleri M.** The current role of erythromycin in the clinical management of gastric emptying disorders. *Am J Gastroenterol.* 1993;88:169–71.

74. **Richards RD, Davenport K, McCallum RW.** The treatment of idiopathic and diabetic gastroparesis with acute intravenous and chronic oral erythromycin. *Am J Gastroenterol.* 1993;88:203–7.

75. **DiBiase JK, Quigley EMM.** Efficacy of prolonged administration of intravenous erythromycin in an ambulatory setting as treatment of severe gastroparesis: one center's experience. *J Clin Gastroenterol.* 1999;28:131–4.

76. **Familoni BO, Abell TL, Voeller G, et al.** Electrical stimulation at a frequency higher than basal rate in human stomach. *Dig Dis Sci.* 1997;42:885–91.

77. **McCallum RW, Chen JDZ, Lin Z, et al.** Gastric pacing improves emptying and symptoms in patients with gastroparesis. *Gastroenterology.* 1998;114:456–61.

78. **Tougas G, Huizinga JD.** Gastric pacing as a treatment for intractable gastroparesis: shocking news? *Gastroenterology.* 1998;114:598–601.

79. **Dobrilla G, Comberlato N, Steela A, Vallaperta P.** Drug treatment of functional dyspepsia: meta-analysis of randomised controlled clinical trials. *J Clin Gastroenterol.* 1989;11:169–77.

80. **Finney JS, Kinnersley N, Hughes M, et al.** Meta-analysis of antisecretory and gastrokinetic compounds in functional dyspepsia. *J Clin Gastroenterol.* 1998;26: 312–20.

81. **Agreus L, Talley NJ.** Challenges in managing dyspepsia in general practice. *BMJ.* 1997;315:1284–8.

82. **Tack J, Broeckaert D, Coulie B, Janssens J.** The influence of cisapride on gastric tone and the perception of gastric distension. *Aliment Pharmacol Ther.* 1998;12: 761–6.

83. **Quigley EMM.** The clinical pharmacology of motility disorder: the perils (and pearls) of prokinesa. *Gastroenterology.* 1994;106:1112–4.

6

■ ■ ■

Dyspepsia and Nonsteroidal Anti-inflammatory Drugs

Walter L. Peterson, MD

Nonsteroidal anti-inflammatory drugs (NSAIDs) are widely used with good effect in patients with rheumatologic disorders, as analgesics in otherwise healthy people, and as prophylaxis against vascular events. Upper gastrointestinal side effects are common with NSAIDs and are a major reason why patients stop taking them. Such side effects include dyspepsia (with or without a co-existing mucosal ulcer) and the more ominous complications of ulceration (bleeding or perforation). Most publications dealing with the side effects of NSAIDs report the "hard" end points of endoscopic ulceration with or without complications. This chapter focuses on the issue of NSAID-related dyspepsia, a much more frequent phenomenon than bleeding or perforation.

Frequency of NSAID-Related Dyspepsia

The lack of a generally accepted definition of dyspepsia has hindered the gathering of accurate data on the prevalence and incidence of dyspepsia in both broad populations and NSAID users. One widely quoted study reported that 62% of patients experienced "dyspepsia" at least once in the previous year, 37% within the previous 2 months, and 29% within the previous week (1). Approximately 15% of patients taking NSAIDs complained of dyspepsia at least once daily for 1 month. These figures may be high because the study's definition of dyspepsia included heartburn (1). The data also suggest that most patients develop symptoms relatively soon after being started on NSAIDs. Perhaps the most reliable data for the prevalence of NSAID-related dyspepsia are found in a meta-analysis of NSAIDs studies published between 1966 and 1997 (2). The authors of this carefully done analysis found that dyspepsia occurred in approximately 2% of placebo-treated patients, rising to 6% to 10% of NSAID-treated patients. These findings are similar to that reported by studies of celecoxib (Celebrex), a new COX-2–selective NSAID, in which over 6000 patients were treated with celecoxib or one of three nonselective NSAIDs. Dyspepsia was reported in 8.8% to 12.8% of patients (Celebrex package insert). Of note, approximately 10% of patients in these studies who developed dyspepsia while taking celecoxib discontinued the medication.

Pathogenesis

Prostaglandin Metabolism

Prostaglandins are formed by the action of cyclooxygenase on arachidonic acid. Recent developments have shown that there are two structurally related isoforms of cyclooxygenase: COX-1 and COX-2. COX-1 is constitutive and is omnipresent in the body, including in the platelets, kidney, and stomach and duodenum (where COX-1–derived prostaglandins presumably mediate normal mucosal integrity) COX-2 is induced by cytokines at sites of injury or autoimmune insult (e.g., joint synovium), where resultant prostaglandin production at least partially meditates inflammation and pain. Drugs that inhibit the expression of COX-2 (e.g., corticosteroids) or the COX-2 mediation of prostaglandin formation (e.g., NSAIDs) also decrease inflammation and pain.

NSAID-Related Gastropathy

Most current NSAIDs nonselectively inhibit both COX-1 and COX-2, thus relieving the inflammation and pain mediated by COX-2–derived prostaglandins while depleting the stomach and duodenum of its COX-1–derived prostaglandins. One consequence of the latter is the formation of gastroduodenal ulceration in some patients. Most of these ulcers are not associated with dyspepsia and are troublesome only if they perforate or breach a major artery, causing it to bleed. The problem of bleeding may be compounded by the fact that COX-1 inhibition also leads to platelet dysfunction. In general, the more COX-1 specific an NSAID is (e.g., indomethacin, ketoprofen), the more ulcerogenic it is; conversely, the less COX-1 specific an NSAID is (e.g., nabumetone, etodolac), the less ulcerogenic it is. However, there are some notable exceptions. For example, ketorolac has a COX-1:COX-2 ratio of close to 1 but is very ulcerogenic. The recognition of the relationship between COX-1 specificity and complications has led to the development of COX-2–selective NSAIDs.

The cause of dyspepsia related to NSAIDs is less clearly understood than the cause of ulceration. Some insight comes from data gathered during the development of COX-2–selective inhibitors, which seem to be as effective as the nonselective NSAIDs in relieving inflammation-induced pain but do not decrease gastric mucosal prostaglandin synthesis as do the nonselective NSAIDs (3). As predicted, clinical studies show that these agents as a group are much less likely to produce gastroduodenal ulceration. However, there is still a substantial incidence of dyspepsia in patients treated with COX-2–selective inhibitors (8.8% with celecoxib vs. 6.2% with placebo) and approximately a 12% incidence with nonselective NSAIDs (Celebrex package insert), suggesting that the depletion of COX-1–derived gastroduodenal prostaglandins is probably not the only cause of dyspepsia. For example, it is possible that both classes of NSAIDs produce microscopic gastroduodenal mucosal damage through topical effects and that such damage predisposes to symptoms.

Relationship of Symptoms to Mucosal Ulceration

There is very poor correlation between dyspepsia and the presence of mucosal ulceration. In one study of 65 patients taking NSAIDs, three of eight patients with dyspepsia had an endoscopic ulcer, whereas only three of 10 patients with an endoscopic ulcer had concomitant symptoms (4). In another study, only 26% of 124 rheumatoid arthritis patients with dyspepsia had ulcers at endoscopy (5).

Management of NSAID-Related Dyspepsia

Stopping or Changing the NSAID

It should go without saying that any patient who develops dyspepsia while taking NSAIDs (especially if there is a clear temporal relationship between the institution of NSAIDs and onset of symptoms) should first reconsider the need for taking the NSAID. If possible, the NSAID should be stopped, a non-NSAID analgesic should be prescribed, and the patient's symptoms should be monitored. If the symptoms resolve, further evaluation is seldom necessary. However, many patients (particularly those with an inflammatory condition for which non-NSAID analgesics are ineffective) will need to continue taking NSAIDs. If this is the case, switching to a different NSAID should be considered, because there is much anecdotal evidence that individual patients who cannot tolerate one NSAID are able to tolerate another without difficulty.

There is much anticipation that the COX-2–selective agents will lead to not only fewer ulcers but also a lower incidence of NSAID-related dyspepsia. Unfortunately, there are no data yet available in peer-reviewed journals either to support or refute such a hypothesis. The package insert for celecoxib (Celebrex), the first COX-2–selective agent to be marketed, suggests that, although there may be slightly fewer symptoms than with nonselective NSAIDs, they are still greater than with placebo.

Endoscopy

Reasons to perform endoscopy in patients taking NSAIDs are shown in Table 6.1. Unless the patient has bled, there is seldom a need for endoscopy. Dyspepsia is a poor predictor of an ulcer, and therapy prescribed to relieve dyspepsia (*see* below) also will treat any ulcer that may be present. Indeed, the primary reason to perform endoscopy on such patients is to find the occasional patient with a gastric malignancy. Simply finding a benign ulcer caused by the NSAID will not change management. This is why the focus of so many NSAID studies on endoscopic ulceration is fallacious. However, it is reasonable to perform endoscopy in patients whose symptoms continue despite cessation of NSAIDs, patients who fail pharmacologic therapy for their dyspepsia, or patients who have alarm symptoms such as weight loss, occult bleeding, or dysphagia.

Pharmacologic Therapy

Patients who must take NSAIDs and whose symptoms persist despite a change in the NSAID may respond to pharmacologic agents that lower gastric acidity. This section focuses only on randomized controlled trials, because open studies of symptoms are notoriously biased. It also should be noted that data on symptom response frequently must be extracted from studies whose primary end point is endoscopic ulcer healing. Al-

---

Table 6.1   Indications for Endoscopy in Patients Taking NSAIDs

- Symptoms continue despite cessation of NSAID

- Symptoms continue despite pharmacologic therapy

- Alarm symptoms (bleeding, weight loss, early satiety) are present

---

though it is not within the scope of this chapter, healing of NSAID-related ulcers with pharmacologic therapy can be summarized as follows: 1) if the NSAID can be stopped, any standard ulcer-healing regimen is effective; 2) if the NSAID cannot be stopped, ulcer healing is best accomplished either with high doses of an H_2-receptor antagonist (H2RA) or with a proton-pump inhibitor (PPI); and 3) duodenal ulcers generally heal more easily than do gastric ulcers.

Antacids

One randomized controlled trial evaluating antacids for the treatment of NSAID-related dyspepsia has been published. Using a small sample size (n = 32), Roth (6) found that mean relief per dose was greater with antacids than with placebo. Unfortunately, actual data were not presented in this abstract and have not been published in a peer-reviewed journal.

Sucralfate

There are no randomized blinded studies assessing sucralfate as a means of relieving NSAID-related dyspepsia.

H_2-Receptor Antagonists

An international randomized controlled trial compared cimetidine 400 mg bid with placebo in 127 patients with ulcer-negative upper abdominal pain who continued to take NSAIDs (7). Upper abdominal pain completely disappeared after 4 weeks in 72% of cimetidine-treated patients compared with 47% of placebo-treated patients (absolute benefit increase [ABI] = 0.25). A second study compared ranitidine 150 mg bid with placebo in 94 arthritis patients with dyspepsia who showed no ulcer at endoscopy (5). After 4 weeks, symptoms were absent in 26% and 6% of ranitidine- and placebo-treated patients, respectively (ABI = 0.20). In summary, acid suppression with H2RAs is effective in relieving NSAID-related upper gastrointestinal symptoms.

Proton-Pump Inhibitors

Two recent studies have compared a PPI (omeprazole) with either ranitidine or misoprostol in patients with NSAID-related ulcers or multiple erosions, some of whom had accompanying dyspepsia. In one study, approximately 50% of patients had moderate to severe dyspepsia on enrollment (8). After 4 weeks, symptoms were moderate to severe in 12% of patients taking ranitidine 150 mg bid and in 6% of patients taking omeprazole 20 mg/d (p = 0.04). At 8 weeks, there were no significant differences. In the companion study, the proportion of patients with moderate to severe symptoms declined from 38% to 11% on misoprostol 200 µg qid and from 45% to 6% on omeprazole 40 mg/d (p = 0.004) (9). These studies evaluated patients with ulcer-associated symptoms; as the ulcers healed, symptoms improved in most patients. There are no studies of PPIs in patients with NSAID-related dyspepsia without ulceration.

Misoprostol

Although there was no placebo group, from the above data it seems that misoprostol reduced NSAID ulcer-related dyspepsia in most patients and only slightly less well than with a PPI (9). This may reflect a beneficial effect of misoprostol on NSAID ulcer healing.

Prophylactic Therapy
To Prevent NSAID-Related Dyspepsia

It is highly unlikely that patients would be given prophylactic therapy that does not protect them from gastroduodenal ulceration as well. Thus, this section assesses the ability to prevent dyspepsia of only those agents reliably proven to prevent NSAID-related ulcers. These are high-dose H2RAs, PPIs, and misoprostol.

Acid Suppression

H$_2$-Receptor Antagonists

In a large trial, arthritis patients without ulceration taking a variety of NSAIDs were randomly assigned for 6 months to placebo, famotidine 20 mg bid, or famotidine 40 mg bid (10). Of note, approximately 30% of patients had "abdominal pain" on entrance into the study. At the end of the study, the absolute decreases in the proportion of patients with abdominal pain were 6%, 7%, and 13%, respectively—a small trend in favor of high-dose famotidine. Of the patients who were symptomatic at the end of the study, it is not known what proportion had symptom-resolution failure or new symptom onset.

Proton-Pump Inhibitors

Two studies have compared omeprazole 20 mg/d with placebo in the prevention of NSAID-related ulceration and onset of new dyspepsia. In the 3-month study (11), 32 of 90 (36%) patients taking placebo developed dyspepsia compared with 13 of 85 (15%) patients taking omeprazole. In the 6-month study (12), 14 of 76 (18%) of placebo-treated patients developed dyspepsia compared with 6 of 75 (8%) patients taking omeprazole. Thus, in each study, there was an approximate 60% reduction in the number of patients experiencing dyspepsia while taking omeprazole compared with placebo.

Misoprostol

Four placebo-controlled studies have assessed the ability of varying doses of misoprostol to prevent NSAID-related ulceration and symptoms (13–16). In no instance was the reported incidence of dyspepsia significantly lower with misoprostol than with placebo. For example, in the very large study of misoprostol in the prevention of ulcer complications, withdrawal for dyspepsia occurred over a 6-month period in 4.6% of patients taking misoprostol compared with 4.1% of patients taking placebo (15).

A double-blind placebo-controlled comparison of misoprostol 200 µg qid and cimetidine 300 mg qid was carried out in 90 previously healthy volunteers given tolmetin 400 mg qid (17). Dyspepsia as an adverse event was noted after 6 days of dosing in 57% of subjects taking placebo, 43% taking misoprostol, and 30% taking cimetidine. In another study comparing misoprostol 200 µg qid with ranitidine 150 mg bid, NSAID-related dyspepsia occurred during an 8-week period in 14% and 10% of patients, respectively (18).

One maintenance-therapy study compared omeprazole 20 mg/d with misoprostol 200 µg bid (9) using the Gastrointestinal Symptom Rating Scale to assess symptoms. Indigestion (not reflux) scores were significantly better with omeprazole than with misoprostol.

Eradication of *Helicobacter pylori*

A large study assessed the development of NSAID-related dyspepsia in patients for 6 months after either the eradication of *Helicobacter pylori* or no eradication (19). Dyspepsia (without ulceration) was noted in 30% of patients after eradication and in 32% of the control group.

Recommendations

- If the evaluation of patients with dyspepsia reveals an ulcer, healing of the ulcer with acid suppression or misoprostol is associated with a resolution of symptoms in most patients. Standard doses of an H2RA or misoprostol are perhaps modestly less effective than a PPI. In patients treated prophylactically, high doses of an H2RA or PPI are superior to misoprostol.

- Eradication of *H. pylori* is not an effective means of preventing NSAID-related dyspepsia.

- The common denominator for maximum effect on dyspepsia seems to be profound acid suppression with either high-dose H2RA or PPI therapy.

■ ■ ■

Key Points

- Most patients who develop NSAID-related dyspepsia do so relatively soon after beginning treatment with NSAIDs.

- In patients using NSAIDs, the correlation between dyspepsia and mucosal ulceration is poor. The first step in the management of NSAID-related dyspepsia involves discontinuation of the NSAID, or, if this is not possible, switching to a different NSAID.

- Endoscopy to identify ulceration is not necessary in patients with NSAID-related dyspepsia; endoscopy is indicated only if gastric cancer is suspected or if symptoms do not resolve with discontinuation of NSAIDs or with pharmacologic therapy.

- Pharmacologic therapy consists of gastric acid suppression with high-dose H2RAs or PPIs.

■ ■ ■

REFERENCES

1. **Larkai EN, Smith JL, Lidsky MD, et al.** Dyspepsia in NSAID users: the size of the problem. *J Clin Gastroenterol.* 1989;11:158–62.

2. **Ofman JJ, Maclean C, Morton S, et al.** The risk of dyspepsia and serious gastrointestinal complications from NSAIDs: a meta-analysis. *Gastroenterology.* In press.

3. **Cryer B, Gottesdiener K, Gertz B, et al.** *In vivo* effects of rofecoxib, a new cyclooxygenase (COX)-2 inhibitor, on gastric mucosal prostaglandin (PG) and serum thromboxane B2 (TXB2) synthesis in healthy humans. *Gastroenterology.* In press.

4. **Larkai EN, Smith JL, Lidsky MD, Graham DY.** Gastroduodenal mucosa and dyspeptic symptoms in arthritic patients during chronic nonsteroidal anti-inflammatory drug use. *Am J Gastroenterol.* 1987;82:1153–7.

5. **Van Groenendael JHLM, Markusse HM, Dijkmans BAC, Breedveld FC.** The effect of ranitidine on NSAID-related dyspeptic symptoms with and without peptic ulcer disease of patients with rheumatoid arthritis and osteoarthritis. *Clin Rheumatol.* 1996;15:450–6.

6. **Roth SH.** Efficacy of antacid therapy for NSAID-induced symptomatic gastropathy (Abstract). *Am J Gastroenterol.* 1993;88:1516.

7. **Bijlsma JWJ.** Treatment of endoscopy-negative NSAID-induced upper gastrointestinal symptoms with cimetidine: an international multicentre collaborative study. *Aliment Pharmacol Ther.* 1988;2S:75–83.

8. **Yeomans ND, Tulassay Z, Juhasz L, et al.** A comparison of omeprazole with ranitidine for ulcers associated with nonsteroidal antiinflammatory drugs. *N Engl J Med.* 1998;338:719–26.

9. **Hawkey CJ, Karrasch JA, Szczepanski L, et al.** Omeprazole compared with misoprostol for ulcers associated with nonsteroidal antiinflammatory drugs. *N Eng J Med.* 1998;338:727–34.

10. **Taha AS, Hudson N, Hawkey CJ, et al.** Famotidine for the prevention of gastric and duodenal ulcers caused by nonsteroidal antiinflamatory drugs. *N Eng J Med.* 1996;334:1435–9.

11. **Ekstrom P, Carling L, Wetterhus S, et al.** Prevention of peptic ulcer and dyspeptic symptoms with omeprazole in patients receiving continuous nonsteroidal anti-inflammatory drug therapy. *Scand J Gastroenterol.* 1996;31:753–8.

12. **Cullen D, Bardhan KD, Eisner M, et al.** Primary gastroduodenal prophylaxis with omeprazole for nonsteroidal anti-inflammatory drug users. *Aliment Pharmacol Ther.* 1998;12:135–40.

13. **Graham DY, Agrawal NM, Roth SH.** Prevention of NSAID-induced gastric ulcer with misprostol: multicentre, double-blind, placebo-controlled trial. *Lancet.* 1988;2:1277–80.

14. **Graham DY, White RH, Moreland LW, et al.** Duodenal and gastric ulcer prevention with misoprostol in arthritis patients taking NSAIDs. *Ann Intern Med.* 1993;119:257–62.

15. **Silverstein FE, Graham DY, Senior JR, et al.** Misoprostol reduces serious gastrointestinal complications in patients with rheumatoid arthritis receiving nonsteroidal anti-inflammatory drugs: a randomized, double-blind, placebo-controlled trial. *Ann Intern Med.* 1995;123:241–9.

16. **Raskin JB, White RH, Jackson JE, et al.** Misoprostol dosage in the prevention of nonsteroidal anti-inflammatory drug-induced gastric and duodenal ulcers: a comparison of three regimens. *Ann Intern Med.* 1995;123:344–50.

17. **Lanza FL, Aspinall RL, Swabb EA, et al.** Double-blind, placebo-controlled endoscopic comparison of the mucosal protective effects of misoprostol versus cimetidine on tolmetin-induced mucosal injury to the stomach and duodenum. *Gastroenterology.* 1988;95:239–94.

18. **Raskin JB, White RH, Jaszewski R, et al.** Misoprostol and ranitidine in the prevention of NSAID-induced ulcers: a prospective, double-blind, multicenter study. *Am J Gastroenterol.* 1996;91:223–7.

19. **Hawkey CJ, Tulassay Z, Szczepanski L, et al.** Randomised controlled trial of *Helicobacter pylori* eradication in patients on nonsteroidal anti-inflammatory drugs: HELP NSAIDs study. *Lancet.* 1998;352:1016–21.

7

Quality-of-Life Issues in Dyspepsia

Kenneth R. DeVault, MD

The term *dyspepsia* has been applied to a variety of symptoms that arise in the upper abdomen and has been suggested to affect up to 25% of the population (1). Dyspepsia may be painful, but it also may be more of a discomfort than a true pain. It is often confused with gastroesophageal reflux disease by both patients and physicians. These complaints are often trivialized as being indigestion or a "functional" disorder.

Quality of life (QOL) refers to aspects that make life worth living and is best reflected in how an individual feels about his or her health and ability to function. Originally a political slogan, QOL was eventually accepted as a scientific concept in the late 1970s. Aspects that are taken into account in QOL determinations include physical function (mobility, self-care), emotional function, social function, role performance (work and home), pain, and disease-specific aspects. The changes of QOL produced by a therapeutic maneuver are important to the lay public, physicians, and policy makers. In diseases without objective markers, QOL may be the best and sometimes only way to measure outcome. In addition, QOL and the general health status of an individual are predictive of medical resource use. A drawback of using QOL is its lack of specificity toward a given symptom or illness. For example, a patient with dyspepsia may achieve complete symptom relief from a trial of an acid blocker, but QOL may not improve appreciably if he or she has other more severe comorbidities (e.g., depression).

A complete discussion of the many instruments used to determine QOL is beyond the scope of this chapter, but there are some excellent reviews available (2). Such instruments must be reliable (i.e., reproducible) and valid (i.e., it measures what it intends to measure). Some questionnaires are designed to be generic, whereas others are disease specific. Commonly used instruments are presented in Table 7.1. Instruments are usually used in research studies; however, because the amount of questioning about general and psychological well-being is often limited in routine practice, there may be a role for these instruments in the clinic. The normal data should be representative of the group of patients studied. Interpreting the subjective end point of dyspepsia can be a source of confusion. Pain and discomfort are mediated by personal experience, cultural values, and other life events, making it difficult to make a comparison of pain responses among many subjects or even in the *same* subject on different days (3). Some evidence indicates that fluctuating levels of endogenous enkephalins may lead to variable intrasubject pain thresholds (4). Finally, the gender and distribution of controls and patients should be similar, because women usually report a lower well-being than do men. In general, well-being also seems to increase with age (5). This variability in the level of well-being between normal groups is especially bothersome in the evaluation of therapeutic changes, which are often difficult to blind to the patient and investigator. This chapter addresses issues related to QOL changes in dyspepsia patients.

Table 7.1   Commonly Used Instruments To Measure Quality of Life

Scale	*Notes*
Karnofsky's Scale (KS)	Developed to measure somatic symptoms in cancer patients
Sickness Impact Profile (SIP)	Commonly used self-reporting scale
Quality of Well-Being Scale (QW-BS)	Sophisticated yet complicated test
Global Assessment of Functioning Scale (GAF)	Well-validated scale that must be administered by a trained interviewer
Psychological General Well-Being Index (PGWB)	Commonly used and self-administered
General Well-Being Schedule (GWB)	Commonly used and self-administered
General Health Questionnaire (GHQ)	Available in 12- to 60-question versions; screens for psychiatric illness.
Gastrointestinal Symptom Rating Scale (GSRS)	Rates gastrointestinal symptoms

Does Dyspepsia Change Quality of Life?

The QOL for dyspepsia patients may be as poor as for patients with somatic diseases, which are usually felt to be more serious. In a study of 1526 patients who presented with symptoms consistent with duodenal ulcer, both the endoscopically positive and negative patients had a low QOL (6). In this large study, the endoscopic findings in the patients with "classic" duodenal ulcer symptoms were esophagitis 13.5%, gastric ulcer 7.7%, duodenal ulcer 29.9%, duodenitis/gastritis 28.2%, and normal 20.8%. QOL was equally affected in each endoscopic category, and almost every measure of QOL was decreased in dyspeptic patients (Fig. 7.1). In a large survey of over 8000 individuals between 40 and 49 years of age, 38% reported symptoms consistent with dyspepsia. These patients had a significantly lower QOL than those without dyspepsia, as measured by the Psychological General Well-Being (PGWB) index (7). Dyspepsia patients had a mean PGWB

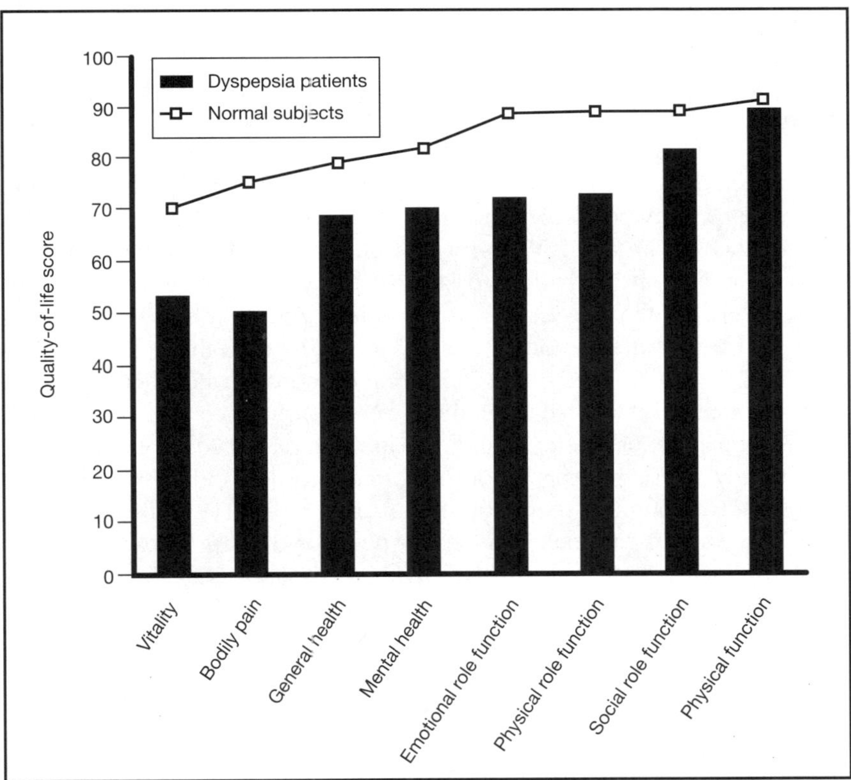

Figure 7.1   Mean health-related quality-of-life scores in patients with at least mild dyspepsia. (Adapted from Wilklund I, Glise H, Jerndal P, et al. Does endoscopy have a positive impact on quality of life in dyspepsia? *Gastrointest Endosc.* 1998;47:449–54.)

index of 98.7 (±15.80) compared with an index of 106.4 (±13.1) in those without dyspepsia ($p < 0.0001$). Dyspepsia resulted in a reduction of 7.27 points in the index when controlled for employment, social class, gender, and other social factors. These patients frequently used antacids and antisecretory medications (43%), and some patients even missed work due to their dyspepsia (2%). In an additional study of 658 patients presenting for endoscopy, the 73 patients with dyspepsia had more impairment in mental health, social functioning, and health perception than did the patients without dyspepsia (8). Although there is currently less emphasis on the subdivision of dyspepsia (e.g., "ulcer-like," "reflux-like," "dysmotility-like"), this study suggested that those with "dysmotility-like" symptoms might have the most impairment in QOL. Gastrointestinal disorders tend to affect QOL more than most other chronic disease states, with exceptions including severe cardiac and psychiatric disease (9). Based on our current understanding, dyspepsia results in a major QOL reduction beyond that produced by many other chronic diseases.

It has been suggested that patients who seek medical attention for upper gastrointestinal symptoms are generally more anxious and distressed than those who do not seek attention and, therefore, have a poor QOL (10). It has even been suggested that up to 60% of patients seen in a gastroenterologist's office may have psychologically based symptoms (11). Factors that have been suggested to contribute to morbidity in patients with dyspepsia include tension, neuroticism, somatization, poor coping skills, and poor support networks (12). This may result in a self-selection process in which patients with anxiety present to a physician and those without anxiety do not. Patients with dyspepsia have been demonstrated to have increased levels of anxiety, tension, hostility, and psychological distress compared with matched normal controls and patients with peptic ulcer disease (13-15). In a detailed study comparing dyspepsia patients with patients with documented duodenal ulcer, there were clearly more depression, anxiety, general psychopathology, and somatization associated with dyspepsia (16). The dyspepsia patients reported more exhaustion and more discomfort in the stomach but also more concerns related to muscle and cardiac pain (Fig. 7.2). There is no clear personality type for dyspepsia, but many patients seem to have difficulty expressing their emotions (alexithymia).

Patients with dyspepsia tend to be younger than patients with peptic ulcer disease. They also are frequently affected at work and are usually less satisfied with the health care system. Both of these factors place negative pressure on QOL. In a large survey of 5430 subjects, 9% of patients with presumed functional gastrointestinal symptoms had missed a mean of 10 work days in the past year (17). Missed workdays due to dyspepsia and many other symptoms seem to correlate with an individual's perception of severity (18). Missing work not only adversely affects an individual's QOL but also negatively affects society as a whole. Dyspepsia can even ad-

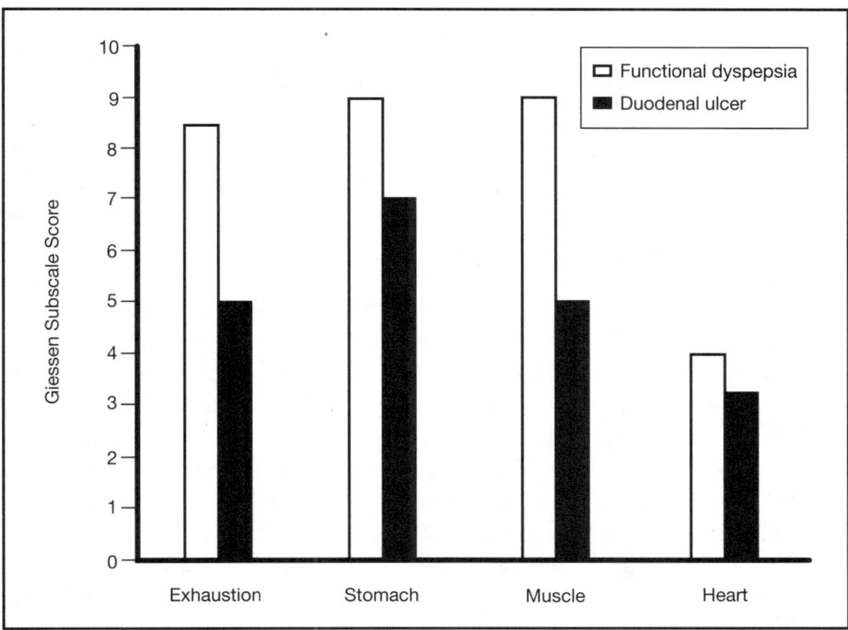

Figure 7.2   Scores on subscales of Giessen Subjective Complaints List for patients with functional dyspepsia or duodenal ulcer. (Adapted from Wilhelmsen I, Haug TT, Ursin H, Berstad A. Discriminant analysis of factors distinguishing patients with functional dyspepsia from patients with duodenal ulcer: significance of somatization. *Dig Dis Sci.* 1995;40:1105–11.)

versely affect sexual function. In a study of 683 patients with dyspepsia and irritable bowel syndrome (IBS) patients, 43.4% reported sexual dysfunction (19). The most common sexual dysfunction was a decrease in sexual drive or desire, and the sexual dysfunction was associated more with symptom severity than with psychological dysfunction. This is probably a nonspecific response to a chronic disease because similar findings have been reported in patients with fibromyalgia and chronic fatigue syndrome. Dyspareunia was seen with IBS, but not with dyspepsia. In addition, dyspareunia has been reported as being due to reflux symptoms that can accompany dyspepsia. These factors all contribute to impaired QOL.

Relationship of Causes of Dyspepsia and Lower Quality of Life

Both sustained activation of the central nervous system and a lowered vagal tone have been postulated as being mechanisms for the association between psychological factors and dyspepsia (20). A Danish study suggested that there is a lower concentration of beta-endorphins in the spinal cord of patients with dyspepsia, but the significance of this finding is unknown (21). Stress itself has been demonstrated to lower the esophageal pain threshold provoked by balloon distention and may also lower the discomfort threshold in dyspepsia (22). Conversely, in a large Australian study, psychological factors (i.e., neuroticism, psychological morbidity, history of abuse) did not seem to be significant predictors for seeking medical attention, whereas symptom severity was predictive (23). Taking all of this information together, it would seem that the decision to seek care for dyspepsia symptoms is multifactorial. Some patients present with severe symptoms, whereas others have symptoms that they feel are severe but that others would find trivial. The latter group's decision to consult may be affected by underlying psychological factors.

It is also possible that dyspepsia represents a reaction to adverse life events and stress that alone can lower QOL. Stressful events have been suggested to increase the risk of both physical and psychological illness (24,25). These stresses and daily hassles also have been correlated with functional abdominal pain and noncardiac chest pain (26,27). A study from Saudi Arabia study reported that individual life-event stresses did not seem to correlate with dyspepsia; however, a Scandinavian study found that patients with dyspepsia had more adverse life events and stress than both normal controls and a matched group of patients with duodenal ulcer (28,29). In the latter study, lower socioeconomic class and a lack of advanced education correlated with both dyspepsia and an increase in adverse life events. Women were more likely to consult than were men. A study from India found more neuroticism but no more stress events (30). Estonian patients with dyspepsia also have an increased incidence of psychoemotional disorders (31). Furthermore, age may be a factor in how an individual responds to dyspepsia. Young patients with dyspepsia tend to have more emotional distress, whereas older patients have more problems with adjustment to vocational, social, and sexual situations (32). It is likely that both the interpretation of and reaction to stress varies between cultures and generations. It is also possible that these cultural factors come into play on QOL determinations. In contrast, an additional study suggested that severity of symptoms, not stressful events, was the only predictive factor of continued problems and impairment in function (33). Thus, even if individuals with dyspepsia seem to have no more stress than would be expected, it seems that they often do not cope well with the stress that they do experience.

Care must be taken when labeling an illness and its resultant affects on QOL as being functional. Although we currently consider nonulcer dyspepsia to be a functional disorder, it is important to note that duodenal ulcer also was considered functional or psychosomatic until recently (34). Perhaps an etiologic factor will be elucidated eventually (as *Helicobacter pylori* has been for ulcer).

Effect of Diagnosis Work-Up on Improving Quality of Life

Dyspepsia patients (and their treating physicians) often have considerable uncertainty about the diagnosis of dyspepsia (35). Up to 40% of those seeking care admit to a fear of underlying malignancy despite its extraordinarily low occurrence in this group (36). The study also found that many patients fear cardiac disease and that the fear of malignancy, cardiac disease, or other serious disease influenced the decision to consult more than the degree of symptoms. Patients from lower social groups tended to have more of these fears and to seek subsequent care. The fear of serious disease is often at least partially related to the nature of the diagnosis. Nonulcer dyspepsia is essentially a diagnosis of exclusion, and there is no study that can provide a positive diagnosis. Despite the fact that patients want to have serious and life-threatening diseases excluded, they often see a series of negative or normal tests as being inconclusive of any specific diagnosis. At times, they tend to think that the best reaction to a negative test is to order more tests, rather than to make a diagnosis based on symptoms and negative testing. More than 90% of patients presenting to physicians with dyspepsia leave the office with a prescription; unfortunately, most studies indicate that little more than a placebo response can be expected from such therapy unless there is a specific pathology (37). When these trials fail, patients frequently experience increased stress and confusion; however, a symptomatic response to therapy gives reassurance to patients in two ways: 1) they feel better, and 2) there is a treatable cause for their symptoms. The consulting patterns and fears of dyspepsia patients are similar to those expressed by IBS patients. In IBS, factors that correlate with health care seeking include frequency and severity of symptoms, visible abdominal distention, anxiety, depression, and fear of the serious nature of their illness (including fear of cancer) (38). Therefore, it is extremely important to address the fears and expectations of these patients in an upfront and caring manner early in the physician-patient interaction.

Simply investigating dyspepsia with a test such as endoscopy may improve QOL by providing more diagnostic information to the patient (39); however, improvement in QOL or patient satisfaction has never been tested in an appropriately designed clinical trial. In one study, endoscopy did not change the gastrointestinal symptoms as measured by the Gastrointestinal Symptoms Rating Scale (2.51 before and 2.42 after endoscopy vs. 1.5 in controls). The overall well-being score (PGWB) did improve (96.8 before and 102.1 after endoscopy, $p < 0.0001$) and approached that of normal controls (102.9). After endoscopy there was also improvement in the ability to perform physical activities and in sleep patterns. Dyspepsia patients with a negative endoscopy have been suggested to have a decrease in their abdominal pain, health care seeking behavior, medication use, and QOL (40,41). In another study, endoscopy usually reassured patients, but there was a subset of patients with a particularly high level of anxiety who had a resurgence of worry and illness belief at 1 month and maintained that worry for at least 1 year (42). Despite trials of medical therapy, most of these patients had persistent symptoms, and subsequently their neuroticism persisted as well. An empirical trial of acid-suppression therapy has been suggested to be unable to provide similar reassurance and improvement in QOL (43). Serologic testing for *H. pylori* with appropriate therapy in those who are positive also may provide reassurance without endoscopy (44).

Improvement in Quality of Life with Therapy Directed at Dyspepsia

Restoration or at least improvement of QOL should be a primary therapeutic goal in dyspepsia and all other diseases. Studies performed on patients with cardiovascular disease suggest a discrepancy between physician- and patient-determined end points (45). Patients are more concerned by the generalized sense of well-being that approximates QOL. A large group of dyspeptic patients ($n = 674$) were randomized to receive either omeprazole or antacids (46). The patients treated with omeprazole were not only more likely to have an improvement in symptoms (64% vs. 30%, $p < 0.0001$) at 4 weeks but also had improvements in their PGWB and Gastrointestinal Symptoms Rating Scale. When a group of patients with severe dyspepsia were treated with either cisapride or domperidone (60-80 mg/d) for 12 months, an improvement in QOL also was found (47). This improvement correlated with the degree of improvement in symptoms and was more profound in patients who initially had more severe symptoms. In another study in which ranitidine was used for patients with documented gastro-esophageal reflux disease, only 24% of patients had a resolution of their symptoms, and improvement in QOL was found only in the subset with improvement (48). If one is seeking to improve QOL, adequate therapy must be offered. For acid-peptic disease, this usually should involve treatment with a proton-pump inhibitor. Although the role of testing for and treating *H. pylori* infection in patients with ulcer-negative dyspepsia is not fully defined, a group of patients with duodenal ulcer and dyspepsia who had their *H. pylori* infection eradicated experienced a return to a normal QOL (49). At 3-year follow-up, the cured patients had better sexual relationships and less psychological distress and exhaustion.

Antinociceptive and psychotropic agents have been used in many functional gastrointestinal disorders. Imipramine and trazodone have been demonstrated to be of benefit in noncardiac chest pain and also have been used in IBS (50,51). The effects of these medications do not seem to be dependent on underlying psychopathology, but no measurement of QOL improvement has been reported. To my knowledge, no randomized trials of this type of therapy in patients with dyspepsia have been published.

Nonpharmacologic therapy also may improve the QOL in patients with dyspepsia. The combination of short-term cognitive therapy and H_2-receptor antagonists resulted in an improvement in QOL in 100 patients with dyspepsia (52). Unfortunately, the improvement did not persist unless therapy was continued, and it was difficult to determine if the psychotherapy had any effect independent of the acid blocker. In the same study, patients with peptic ulcer disease also had normalization of QOL after eradication of *H. pylori*, and this improvement in QOL did persist after therapy.

Conclusions

It is clear that dyspepsia is a symptom complex that produces anxiety and impairs QOL. The improvement of both diagnostic certainty (i.e., ruling out other more "serious" diseases) and symptoms improve QOL in many, if not most, patients. When a specific etiologic factor is discovered (e.g., ulcer disease, esophagitis), proper therapy not only controls that factor but also restores QOL. Although the causal relationship between stress and dyspepsia (and vice versa) is debatable, their interaction is indisputable. A successful consultant should address stress and many other factors when confronted with a dyspepsia patient. These factors may include anxiety, tension, neuroticism, somatization, fear of malignancy or heart disease, history of sexual abuse, and many other potential physical and psychological issues. This approach results in an improvement in symptoms and QOL in many patients.

Key Points

- QOL for patients with dyspepsia may be as poor as (or poorer than) that for patients with a more serious disease.

- Dyspepsia has been shown to result in a mean of 10 missed work days per year; sexual dysfunction; and increased levels of anxiety, depression, and somatization.

- Diagnostic evaluation for the causes of dyspepsia may in itself improve QOL when the diagnosis offers reassurance that serious or fatal disease is not present.

- Improvement in QOL should be one of the primary goals of dyspepsia management.

REFERENCES

1. **Talley NJ, Zinsmeister AR, Schleck CD, Meton LJ III.** Dyspepsia and dyspepsia subgroups: a population-based study. *Gastroenterology.* 1992;102:1259–68.

2. **Dimenas E, Carlsson G, Glise H, et al.** Relevance of norm values as part of the documentation of quality-of-life instruments for use in upper gastrointestinal disease. *Scand J Gastroenterol.* 1996;31(Suppl 221):8–13.

3. **Wolff BB.** Behavioral measurements of human pain. In Steinbach RA (ed). *The Psychology of Pain.* New York: Raven Press; 1978:129–68.

4. **McGivern RF, Berntson GG.** Mediation of diurnal fluctuations in pain sensitivity in the rat by food intake patterns: reversal by Naloxone. *Science.* 1980;210:210–1.

5. **Tibblin G, Bengtsson C, Furunes B, et al.** Symptoms by age and sex: the population studies of men and women in Gothenburg Sweden. *Scand J Prim Health Care.* 1990;8:9–17.

6. **Dimenas E, Glise H, Hallerback B, et al.** Well-being and gastrointestinal symptoms among patients referred to endoscopy owing to suspected duodenal ulcer. *Scand J Gastroenterol.* 1995;30:1046–52.

7. **Moayyedi P.** *Clinical and Economic Impact of Dyspepsia in the Community.* Paper presentation at the pH-Hp Implications for Dyspepsia Management, Geneva, Switzerland, 1998.

8. **Talley NJ, Weaver AL, Zinmeister AR.** Impact of functional dyspepsia on quality of life. *Dig Dis Sci.* 1995;40:584–9.

9. **Stewart AL, Greenfield S, Hays RD, et al.** Functional status and well-being of patients with chronic conditions: results from the medical outcomes study. *JAMA.* 1989;262:907–13.

10. **Johnston BT, Gunning J, Lewis SA.** Health care seeking by heartburn sufferers is associated with psychosocial factors. *Am J Gastroenterol.* 1996;91:2500–4.

11. **Folks DG, Kinny FC.** The role of psychological factors in gastrointestinal conditions: a review pertinent to DSM-IV. *Psychosomatics.* 1992;33:257–70.

12. **Wilklund I, Butler-Wheelhouse P.** Psychosocial factors and their role in symptomatic gastroesophageal reflux disease and functional dyspepsia. *Scand J Gastroenterol.* 1996;220(Suppl):94–100.

13. **Jonsson BH, Theorell T, Gotthard R.** Symptoms and personality in patients with chronic functional dyspepsia. *J Psychosom Res.* 1995;39:93–102.

14. **Langeluddecke P, Goulston K, Tennant C.** Psychological factors in dyspepsia of unknown cause: a comparison with peptic ulcer. *J Psychosom Res.* 1990;34:215–22.

15. **Wilhelmsen I, Bakke A, Tangen Haug T, et al.** Psychosocial Adjustment to Illness Scale (PAIS-SR) in a Norwegian material of patients with functional dyspepsia, duodenal ulcer, and urinary bladder dysfunction: clinical validation of the instrument. *Scand J Gastroenterol.* 1994;29:611–7.

16. **Wilhelmsen I, Haug TT, Ursin H, Berstad A.** Discriminant analysis of factors distinguishing patients with functional dyspepsia from patients with duodenal ulcer: significance of somatization. *Dig Dis Sci.* 1995;40: 1105–11.

17. **Drossman DA, Li Z, Andruzzi E, et al.** U.S. householder survey of functional gastrointestinal disorders: prevalence, sociodemography, and health impact. *Dig Dis Sci.* 1993;38:1569–80.

18. **Nyren O, Adami HO, Gustavsson S, Loof L.** Excess sick-listing in nonulcer dyspepsia. *J Clin Gastroenterol.* 1986;8:339–45.

19. **Fass R, Fullerton S, Naliboff B, et al.** Sexual dysfunction in patients with irritable bowel syndrome and nonulcer dyspepsia. *Digestion.* 1998;59:79–85.

20. **Tangen Haug T, Svebak S, Hausken T, et al.** Low vagal activity as mediating mechanism for the relationship between personality factors and gastric symptoms in functional dyspepsia. *Psychosom Med.* 1994;56:181–6.

21. **Jorgneson LS, Bach FW, Christiansen PM, et al.** Reduced concentration of beta-endorphin in cerebrospinal fluid and reduced pain tolerance in patients with functional dyspepsia. *Ugeskr Laeger.* 199;157:166–9.

22. **Anderson KO, Dalton CB, Bradley LA, Richter JE.** Stress induces alteration of esophageal pressures in healthy volunteers and noncardiac chest pain patients. *Dig Dis Sci.* 1989;34:83–91.

23. **Talley NJ, Boyce P, Jones M.** Dyspepsia and health care seeking in a community: How important are psychological factors? *Dig Dis Sci.* 1998;43:1016–22.

24. **Rabkin J, Stuening E.** Life events, stress, and illness. *Science.* 1976;194:1013–20.

25. **Brown GW, Harris T.** *Social Origins of Depression.* London: Tavistock, 1978.

26. **Creed F, Craig T, Armer RJ.** Functional abdominal pain, psychiatric illness, and life events. *Gut.* 1988;29:235–42.

27. **Lau GK, Hui WM, Lam SK.** Life events and daily hassles in patients with atypical chest pain. *Am J Gastroenterol.* 1996;91:2157–62.

28. **Hafeiz HB, al-Quorain A, al Mangoor S, Karim AA.** Life events stress in functional dyspepsia: a case-control study. *Eur J Gastroenterol Hepatol.* 1997;9:21–6.

29. **Haug TT, Wilhelmsen I, Berstad A, Ursin H.** Life events and stress in patients with functional dyspepsia compared with patients with duodenal ulcer and healthy controls. *Scand J Gastroenterol.* 1995;30:524–30.

30. **Jain Ak, Gupta JP, Gupta S, et al.** Neuroticism and stressful life events in patients with nonulcer dyspepsia. *J Assoc Phys India.* 1195;43:90–1.

31. **Lond E, Varmann P, Elshtein N, et al.** Dyspepsia in rural residents of Estonia: life-style factors, psychoemotional disorders, and familial history of gastrointestinal diseases. *Scand J Gastroenterol.* 1995;30:826–8.

32. **Wilhelmsen I, Bakke A, Tangen Haug T, et al.** Psychosocial adjustment to illness scale in a Norwegian material of patients with functional dyspepsia, duodenal ulcer, and urinary bladder dysfunction: clinical validation of the instrument. *Scand J Gastroenterol.* 1994;29:611–7.

33. **Talley NJ, McNeil D, Hayden A, et al.** Prognosis of chronic unexplained dyspepsia: a prospective study of potential predictor variables in patents with endoscopically diagnosed nonulcer dyspepsia. *Gastroenterology.* 1987;92:1060–6.

34. **Alexander F.** *Psychosomatic Medicine: Its Principles and Applications.* New York: WW Norton; 1950.

35. **Heatley RV, Rathbone BJ.** Dyspepsia: dilemma for doctors. *Lancet.* 1987;2:779–82.

36. **Lydeard S, Jones R.** Factors affecting the decision to consult with dyspepsia: comparison of consulters and nonconsulters. *J R Coll Gen Pract.* 1989;39:495–8.

37. **Veldhuyzen van Zanten AJO, Cleary C, Talley NJ, et al.** Drug treatment of functional dyspepsia: a systematic analysis of trial methodology with recommendations for design of future trials. *Am J Gastroenterol.* 1996;91:660–73.

38. **Kettell J, Jones R, Lydeard S.** Reasons for consultation in irritable bowel syndrome: symptoms and patients characteristics. *Br J Gen Pract.* 1992;42:459–61.

39. **Wilklund I, Glise H, Jerndal P, et al.** Does endoscopy have a positive impact on quality of life in dyspepsia. *Gastrointest Endosc.* 1998;47:449–54.

40. **Talley NJ, McNeil D, Hayden A, et al.** Prognosis of chronic unexplained dyspepsia. *Gastroenterology.* 1987;92:1060–6.

41. **Jones R.** What happens to patients with nonulcer dyspepsia after endoscopy? *Practitioner.* 1988;232:75–8.

42. **Lucock MP, Morley S, White C, et al.** Responses of consecutive patients to reassurance after gastroscopy: results of self-administered questionnaire survey. *BMJ.* 1997;315:572–5.

43. **Betyxer P, Moller Hansen J, Schafalitzky de Muckadell OB.** Empirical H_2-blocker therapy of prompt endoscopy in management of dyspepsia. *Lancet.* 1994;343:811–6.

44. **Patel P, Khulusi S, Mendall MA, et al.** Prospective screening of dyspeptic patients by *Helicobacter pylori* serology. *Lancet.* 1995;346:1315–8.

45. **Wiklund I, Comerford B, Dimenas E.** The relationship between exercise tolerance and quality of life in angina pectoris. *Clin Cardiol.* 1991;14:204–8.

46. **Groves J, Oldring JK, Kerr D, et al.** First line treatment with omeprazole provides an effective and superior alternative strategy in the management of dyspepsia compared to antacid/alginate liquid: a multicentre study in general practice. *Aliment Pharmacol Ther.* 1998;12:147–57.

47. **Cutts TF, Abell TL, Karas JG, Kuns J.** Symptom improvement from prokinetic therapy corresponds to improved quality of life in patients with severe dyspepsia. *Dig Dis Sci* 1996;41:1369–78.

48. **Revicki DA, Wood M, Maton PN, Sorensen S.** The impact of gastroesophageal reflux disease on health-related quality of life. *Am J Med.* 1998;104:252–8.

49. **Wilhelmsen I.** Quality of life and *Helicobacter pylori* eradication. *Scand J Gastroenterol.* 1996;221(Suppl):18–20.

50. **Cannon RO, Quyyumi AA, Mincemoyer R, et al.** Imipramine in patients with chest pain despite normal coronary angiograms. *N Engl J Med.* 1994,330:1411–7.

51. **Clouse RE, Lustman PJ, Eckert TC, et al.** Low-dose trazodone for symptomatic patients with esophageal contraction abnormalities: a double-blind placebo-controlled trial. *Gastroenterology.* 1987;92:1027–36.

52. **Wilhelmsen I.** Quality of life in upper gastrointestinal disorders. *Scand J Gastroenterol.* 1995;211(Suppl):21–5.

8

Clinical and Economic Effects of Nonprescription Therapy in the Treatment of Dyspepsia

A. Mark Fendrick, MD

This chapter provides an overview of the social, clinical, and economic considerations that underlie the common decision by individuals with dyspepsia to use nonprescription therapy and to defer medical consultation. The potential advantages and risks associated with self-treatment of dyspepsia are discussed. Given the positive clinical and economic expectations that accompanied the availability of nonprescription H_2-receptor antagonists (H2RAs), a review of the available evidence is presented.

Background

Because the definition of dyspepsia varies in community-based epidemiologic investigations, published prevalence values range from 13% to 40% (1–3); because symptoms seem to come and go, the calculation of the actual incidence of dyspepsia is somewhat problematic (3). Despite the high prevalence and access to numerous diagnostic and treatment modalities, an incomplete understanding of the pathophysiology of dyspepsia persists. These limitations, together with an inability to correlate observed symptoms to identified abnormalities on diagnostic testing (4,5), have generated significant and long-standing controversy about the optimal clinical management of dyspepsia (6). Most individuals with dyspepsia symptoms (~75%) do not seek medical attention (7), and little attention has been paid to why symptomatic individuals do not formally seek medical care (although one study has addressed the reasons for seeking a medical consultation for dyspepsia once the decision to seek care has been made [8]). Hypotheses explaining the decision to defer care include the minimal effect of symptoms on quality of life, the availability of effective nonprescription therapy, a lack of concern or ignorance of potentially serious yet treatable underlying conditions, and a lack of awareness of more effective treatment options.

It remains unclear whether users of nonprescription therapies are well informed of the potential risks of self-therapy or the availability of potentially more effective pharmaceutical alternatives. Direct-to-consumer campaigns sponsored by professional medical societies and pharmaceutical manufacturers have been undertaken to improve the knowledge of the lay public regarding these issues. Although the initial response (as measured by first-time calls to toll-free telephone hotlines) has been impressive (American College of Gastroenterology, Unpublished data), the effect of these educational campaigns on physician visits, drug use, diagnostic testing, and most importantly patient satisfaction has not been reported.

Abdominal symptoms are the primary complaint for an estimated 2% to 4% of primary care office visits (5,7). However, a visit to a physician for another reason does not guarantee that dyspepsia symptoms will be raised by the patient and addressed adequately. A recent telephone survey of 2000 individuals with heartburn reported that 199 of 815 (21%) with frequent symptoms and 566 of 1058 (53%) with infrequent symptoms did not inform their physician about their heartburn (9). Regression modeling revealed that increasing age, female sex, higher education level, and frequency of symptoms were significant predictors of reporting behavior. If contact with the health care system can provide an additional element of clinical value to individuals with dyspepsia, both patients and physicians must ensure that information about these symptoms is properly conveyed.

For reasons that have been only partially explained, nonprescription drug therapy is the first and most common type of treatment used for the great majority of dyspepsia patients (10). A recent community-based survey of individuals with heartburn reported that more than 75% took a nonprescription medication for their symptoms (9). Why an individual chooses to use prescription drugs, as opposed to nonprescription agents, has not been well studied. One epidemiologic investigation of a community-resident elderly population identified that prescription drug use (compared with nonprescription drug use) was best predicted by previous use, older age, white race, poorer health, and number of health care visits, suggesting that more attention is needed to ensure equitable access to prescription agents (11).

When the decision to use nonprescription therapy is made, there is a paucity of information in the literature addressing how an individual chooses among the numerous nonprescription therapies available for dyspeptic symptoms. The potential merits of all types of agents are aggressively advertised directly to consumers in the print, radio, and television media. There is tremendous variation in mechanism of action (e.g., antigas, stomach coating, antacid), onset of relief (e.g., prophylaxis, rapid relief, long-acting relief), formulations (e.g., liquids, chewable tablets, pills), and cost among the available agents. Despite these differences and the widespread use of all of these therapies, controlled head-to-head investigations to assess the relative effectiveness and cost effectiveness in unselected dyspepsia patients have not been, and are unlikely to be, performed. Thus, it seems that once the decision to use a nonprescription dyspepsia agent is made, the choice of a specific over-the-counter (OTC) therapy is more likely to be made on nonscientific (e.g., word of mouth, marketing, out-of-pocket cost) than on scientific grounds.

Prescription Therapies Made
Available as Over-the-Counter Treatments

In the past decade, a new class of nonprescription pharmaceutical agents has become available. The number of these drugs—either at prescription strength or a lower dose—is expected to continue to rise (12). There are social and economic forces behind this trend. Social considerations include the increasing desire of people to have a greater level of input into seeking medical care services. Such a philosophy assumes that individuals want more autonomy in their health care and that they will take an increasing responsibility for it. Access to these agents is based on a premise that the benefits achieved exceed the risks incurred in both individual patients and the total population. There is significant debate among patients, clinicians, and government regulators as to whether these empowering attributes are justified given the attendant risks of self-treatment (13).

For a prescription product to be approved for OTC use, new and separate clinical studies must pass the scrutiny of the Food and Drug Administration (FDA). Although this safeguard is an important one, there are many differences between controlled clinical investigations (i.e., a restricted range of patients under controlled conditions) and an uncontrolled community environment. This concern is highlighted by the fact that postmarketing surveillance studies are often poorly planned and executed. Thus, demonstrating a convincing safety profile at OTC doses is paramount for approval because of the potential for errors in self-diagnosis or drug use. Given how quickly prescription drugs are moving to the nonprescription sector, clinicians must pay close attention to whether there are sufficient mechanisms in place to detect inappropriate use and unexpected adverse events. At present, the clinical benefits are more easily tallied than the risks, whose true burden is difficult, if not impossible, to quantify.

The rapid push to make more prescription drugs available OTC may be based more on economic forces than on social factors. After a brief respite in the growth rate of health care costs in the mid-1990s, double-digit increases in medical expenditures have resumed, fueled significantly by the increased use of pharmaceuticals. Although pharmaceutical expenditures represent the fastest-growing sector of health care delivery, they also represent the greatest opportunity for reducing morbidity and mortality and for enhancing cost-effective and, in rare instances, cost-*saving* medical care. Encouraging individuals to purchase nonprescription pharmaceuticals directly without (and sometimes with) the advice of a clinician can constrain overall drug spending or, at minimum, transfer the economic burden of increasing pharmaceutical sales from the health payer to the patient.

Cost savings attributable to the switch of a prescription drug to OTC status was demonstrated in a managed care setting by Gurwitz and coworkers (14). Data from a northeastern United States health plan were used, and the introduction of nonprescription vaginal antifungal products was the model. Comparing the years before and after the introduction of OTC vaginal antifungal agents, they reported significant decreases in physician visits and prescriptions for vaginitis after only 1 year of OTC availability. They concluded that the cost savings attributable to an OTC switch can occur in a managed care setting. However, they appropriately noted that these favorable effects on costs needed to be weighed against the shift of cost to consumers and the potential adverse events that may result from errors in self-diagnosis.

As a result, managed care organizations are encouraging self-care with nonprescription drugs. One group-model health maintenance organization has implemented a program to target alternative nonprescription agents that may be substituted for prescription drugs (15). Patient satisfaction, resource-use reductions, and education are the stated goals. The hypotheses are that the promotion of self-care can decrease visits with physicians and nurses, reduce phone communication, and lower pharmacist workload for prescriptions. In this program, pharmacists are actively involved to ensure the safe and effective use of nonprescription agents through the use of educational displays and counseling.

There are few published data on patient attitudes toward a physician recommending self-care with nonprescription drugs. A recently published survey of 2765 patients in Birmingham, United Kingdom, reported attitudes toward physicians inquiring about and recommending OTC agents (16). Half of the respondents took regularly prescribed medications, and one quarter used nonprescription drugs. The patients were positive toward physicians inquiring about OTC drug use. They also welcomed physicians making nonprescription recommendations, especially in those rare instances in which the OTC agents cost less than the insurance co-pay. However, patients responded negatively to the idea that pharmacists should play a more significant role in making therapeutic decisions.

From the physician's perspective, it seems that, in the absence of any clear financial incentives to reduce drug expenditures (at a cost of lower patient satisfaction), they will be unlikely to recommend a switch from prescription to OTC agents. A recent survey of general practitioners in London reported that 54% of responders supported the use of OTC H2RAs for patients under 45 years of age who had not responded to antacids (17). Despite this apparent vote of confidence for OTC H2RAs, the responding general practitioners noted that they had barely changed their prescribing patterns since these agents became available in nonprescription form.

Interestingly, even for those doctors who have a financial stake in pharmaceutical costs, reduced expenditures in drugs may not be worth the time it takes to consult a patient about a switch from a prescription to an OTC drug. One clinical practice in the United Kingdom estimated that a net savings of less than 1% would result from an aggressive strategy switching patients from prescription to OTC drugs (18). When asked about the potential growing role of pharmacists in the OTC strategy, nearly 50% of physicians expressed some concern about a patient going to a pharmacist for advice about a pharmaceutical therapy.

Nonprescription H$_2$-Receptor Antagonists as Over-the-Counter Treatments

The approval of nonprescription H2RAs for consumer purchase was met with great fanfare by patients and health care payers. For all OTC H2RA preparations, the nonprescription dose was one half the standard prescription dose. Direct-to-consumer advertisements heralding the OTC switch were distributed rapidly and widely in an attempt to ensure consumer knowledge of their availability. For individuals who are less likely to try the product, direct-mail samples and price-discount coupons were made plentiful to encourage an initial trial.

There were high expectations that many individuals with dyspepsia who were not taking prescription agents would receive a significant improvement in symptom relief compared with previously available OTC products. The convenience associated with the ability to purchase a familiar, safe, and effective agent was welcomed by users of OTC agents. Furthermore, because all four H2RAs available by prescription (cimetidine, ranitidine, famotidine, and nizatidine) rapidly received FDA approval for their lower-dose nonprescription forms, individuals who previously required a prescription from a health care provider could now purchase their preferred product without one.

At one time, H2RAs were the world's most prescribed and most costly class of pharmaceuticals. When they became available in nonprescription formulations, economic benefits to health care payers were anticipated. It was hoped that the relative reductions of physician visits, diagnostic procedures, and prescription pharmaceuticals would be similar to those achieved when OTC vaginal antifungal agents became available (14). Because the absolute number of visits for dyspepsia and expenditures for antisecretory agents far outnumbered visits and drug costs for vaginitis, a similar rate of reduction in these resources would have signified a welcome and marked decrease in overall health care costs. Any effect on prescription drug costs would be particularly important in the case of dyspepsia. A claims database study examining data on health care use among Pennsylvania Medicaid enrollees with dyspepsia found that 75% of costs of dyspepsia ($51 of $68 per month) were accounted for by drugs (19). From a social perspective, added economic benefits from improved therapy were supposed to occur as a result of an expected reduction in dyspepsia-related productivity losses. A 1998 survey of dyspepsia patients in the Netherlands reported that 38% of respondents were absent an average of 1.9 days from work because of dyspepsia-related symptoms during the previous 4 weeks (20).

When OTC H2RAs became available, Oster and coworkers (21) constructed a decision-analysis model that estimated the clinical and economic effects of the availability of nonprescription H2RAs. The simulation projected that, because of the widespread use of OTC agents, the number of people seeking professional care for dyspepsia would decrease by over 1 million per year, with the attendant decreases in prescription medications (21). Another published decision analysis by Kalish and coworkers (22) was less confident that significant cost savings would be achieved by a managed care organization resulting from the OTC switch. Their analysis suggested that the cost savings attributable to decreased prescription drug use would be offset by a possible increase in diagnostic testing related to treatment failures with nonprescription H2RAs.

Dyspepsia and Nonprescription Therapy

Dyspepsia is a common clinical condition that is well suited to highlighting the dynamics of a changing health care delivery system that allows symptomatic individuals a great deal of choice when it comes to the decision about whether to self-treat or seek medical advice. The symptomatic patient is central to the decision because there is a clear option of seeking potentially effective care with or without the need of formal medical consultation.

If an individual chooses to seek professional care within the health care system, the patient also has the option of seeing a primary care provider or a subspecialist. In instances of severe symptoms or complications, he or she may report to an emergency room or hospital. Depending on the option chosen, the individual patient may experience significant financial (depending on presence and type of insurance coverage) and nonfinancial (e.g., waiting time for appointments) consequences. In a great majority of cases, the first interaction with the health care system is with a primary care provider. However, it is not unusual that the initial physician consulted for persistent or severe abdominal symptoms is a gastroenterologist or surgeon.

Predictors for Seeking Medical Care

The decision to seek medical attention for a bothersome symptom is complicated and often based on symptom type, severity, and duration (23). In circumstances in which the symptom is common, mild or moderate in severity, and/or believed not to be associated with a poor clinical outcome, the desire to seek care may not be great. The option of purchasing potentially effective therapy without the need for a prescription is also an important factor that influences the decision to visit a health professional. Access to therapy that is effective in decreasing or eliminating the symptom is a welcome option, because it provides an individual autonomy as to choice of therapy and whether or not treatment should be initiated (or continued).

For many individuals, the decision to visit a health care professional may be related to nonclinical factors such as distance, availability of transportation, scheduling, or access to health insurance. Yet individuals with health insurance still may defer a visit to a health professional due to anxiety, concerns over out-of-pocket expenditures, or expectations of the physician visit.

From their study of determinants to seek a physicians' care, Wagner and coworkers (23) suggest that there are clear differences in the determinants to seek care for nonsevere symptoms among frequent users of medical services than among infrequent users. Somewhat surprisingly, the results demonstrated that frequent users of physician services do not necessarily treat themselves more frequently with nonprescription medications when compared with the infrequent users. These data suggest that those who seek physician care frequently have an altered perception of the physician's role and have different expectations of a health care consultation.

Nonprescription Treatment of Dyspepsia

Antacids and H2RAs are the drugs most commonly used to relieve symptoms of dyspepsia. In a great majority of instances, the primary outcome desired by patients with dyspepsia is symptom relief. Another significant concern elicited from patients seeking medical attention for dyspepsia is anxiety about underlying diagnosis (8). Given the explicit and implicit trade-offs between the decision to seek or avoid formal medical therapy for dyspepsia symptoms, an improved understanding of the different benefits, risks, and costs between self-treatment and professional consultation is needed.

The nonprescription treatment options currently available for dyspepsia are numerous. The required regulatory requirements demonstrating the safety and efficacy of these products vary depending on the type of product. OTC pharmaceutical agents must demonstrate safety and efficacy for specific indications to receive approval by the FDA. Vitamins, herbal products, and nutritional supplements are not required to undergo similar rigorous scrutiny before they are permitted to enter the marketplace.

Lifestyle Modification

Lifestyle and dietary modification to eliminate inciting factors or to alter underlying pathophysiology are frequently recommended to dyspepsia patients. There are no controlled investigations of lifestyle modification for patients with uninvestigated dyspepsia. For patients with gastroesophageal reflux disease, studies have demonstrated that decreasing dietary fat, elevating the head of the bed, and avoiding a recumbent posture will decrease esophageal acid exposure (24). Although it is wise to recommend that a patient stop smoking or lose weight if obese, it is unclear that an improvement in dyspepsia symptoms will result.

For obvious reasons, compliance with lifestyle modifications is not overwhelmingly high. Even when certain foods and lifestyles are identified as being potential causes of heartburn, most patients do not modify these behaviors (9). The lack of apparent effectiveness can be seen in the actions of physicians. Less than 50% of patients with gastroesophageal reflux disease report that their physicians had discussed most of the recommended lifestyle modifications, which suggests a lack of confidence in their usefulness (25). However, physicians are likely to modify their lifestyle advice based on specific patient characteristics.

Herbal Preparations

Herbal preparations have long been used to treat dyspepsia, despite a lack of evidence for their use. Recently, a double-blind placebo-controlled trial was performed comparing iberogast (a combination of bitter candy tuft, *Matricaria* flower, peppermint, caraway, licorice root, and *Melissa* balm) with placebo, in patients with nonulcer dyspepsia (26). Enrolled patients (*n* = 118) had symptoms for an average of 7 years. At 4 weeks, 78% of patients treated with the herbal preparation had improvements in symptoms compared with 39% in the placebo arm. At 8 weeks, 20% of the iberogast-treated patients were completely free of symptoms. Treatment with ibero-gast seemed to have an effect on sick leave for dyspeptic symptoms; only 4% reported taking sick leave while taking iberogast compared with 28% taking placebo.

Antacids

Antacids are extensively used nonprescription agents; they are inexpensive, fast acting, and available in a number of different forms. Antacids increase the pH of gastric contents, deactivate pepsin, and may prevent reflux by increasing lower esophageal sphincter pressure. Despite their widespread use, no formal studies comparing antacids to other nonprescription agents for the treatment of dyspepsia have been undertaken. Data became available only when antacids were used as a control in trials of low-dose prescription agents. For patients with nonulcer dyspepsia, controlled studies revealed that antacids provided little benefit (27). One controlled trial from the United Kingdom randomized uninvestigated patients with dyspepsia to receive either antacids or omeprazole 10 mg every morning for 4 weeks (28). Omeprazole was found to be statistically superior to antacids for all end points. At 4 weeks, antacids achieved complete relief of heartburn (the most common symptom at entry) in 30% of patients (omeprazole 64%) and complete relief of overall symptoms in 16% (omeprazole 41%). Uncontrolled epidemiologic investigations suggest that these agents are often used successfully in patients who self-medicate for reflux symptoms (29). Although antacids may be effective in providing short-term relief of heartburn, they are probably not effective in healing esophagitis (29).

A 1986 study of low-risk dyspepsia patients demonstrated that 3 weeks of high-dose antacid therapy led to a considerable improvement in 68% of patients (30). As a result of the clinical improvement, there was a significant decrease in requests for upper gastrointestinal radiography by patients and physicians. This change in ordering behavior for diagnostic testing led to a 37% reduction in charges. No complications were detected after 18 months of follow-up. These results suggest that improvement in symptoms confer reassurance to such an extent that a diagnostic investigation to determine the underlying cause of the symptoms may be deferred or eliminated.

Antacids may be effective in providing symptom relief, but when used at high doses, as described in the study above, they can cause adverse effects such as fluid retention, milk-alkali syndrome, and alterations in lower gastrointestinal function (e.g. constipation, diarrhea). At high doses, they also have the potential to produce drug interactions by altering drug binding or changing gastric pH, which affects drug absorption.

Nonprescription H$_2$-Receptor Antagonists

All four OTC H2RAs (cimetidine, ranitidine, famotidine, and nizatidine) are effective in self-directed treatment for intermittent heartburn. In one study, OTC famotidine was also effective in preventing food-induced symptoms, thus justifying its prophylactic claim (31). Antacids, which were used as a control, were also found to be effective. Both treatments were equally well tolerated.

Have the OTC H2RAs lived up to the expectations of more symptom relief, fewer physician visits, and lower prescription drug costs for individuals with dyspepsia? Few available data address this question. Gurwitz and colleagues (14) studied the effect of the availability of OTC H2RAs on prescribing patterns and physician visits among a group of chronic prescription H2RA users. Over a 1-year period, the mean number of prescription H2RAs was reduced by 1.5 per person. There was a slightly lower reduction with all gastrointestinal agents, suggesting that a small portion of the overall decrease was due to a shift to other prescription products. There was no reported decrease in physician visits.

A recent community-based survey to determine the effects of OTC H2RAs in dyspepsia patients demonstrated that only 15% of regular OTC users achieved complete symptom relief (32). From self-reports of care-seeking behavior, the expected cost savings due to the reduction of physician visits did not occur. These studies—one in patients most likely to demonstrate a reduction in drug costs (chronic prescription H2RA users) and the other in patients most likely to defer physician visits (OTC users)—suggest that the large anticipated savings to payers is unlikely to occur.

Risks of Nonprescription Therapy in Dyspepsia

Despite the empowering aspects associated with the self-treatment of dyspeptic symptoms, there are downside risks. Some of the more serious shortcomings of the use of nonprescription therapy include missing serious diagnoses and delaying access to necessary or superior treatments.

Drug Side Effects and Interactions

Among the risks generally associated with OTC treatment are drug-related side effects, drug interactions, and inappropriate treatment. However, nearly two decades of evidence assessing the safety of the four available H2RAs (cimetidine, ranitidine, famotidine, and nizatidine) suggest that this class of pharmaceuticals is among the safest known. The agents are well tolerated, with a low overall incidence of drug-related adverse effects. The most common drug interactions occur with cimetidine when taken with meperidine, theophylline, warfarin, ketoconazole, or oral hypoglycemics.

Missed Diagnoses

The potential for nonprescription medication to mask serious illness is a significant concern. It was not until recently that appropriately designed investigations were undertaken to provide information addressing this important issue. In 1998, Robinson and coworkers (33) identified, through community-based advertisements, 178 otherwise healthy adults who had a history of heartburn relieved by antacids (for at least 3 months) *and* who experienced heartburn on at least 4 of the 7 days before study entry (33). Patients were excluded if a previous diagnostic study was performed. The mean duration of heartburn was 11 years, and nearly 50% of patients had daily heartburn during the previous year, suggesting severe disease. Twenty-two individuals were discovered to have major disease after diagnostic testing: nondysplastic Barrett's esophagus (n = 9), esophageal spasm (n = 7), peptic ulcer disease (n = 4), dysplastic Barrett's esophagus (n = 1), and Barrett's esophagus with cancer (n = 1). Erosive esophagitis was present in nearly half of the remaining patients, although only two-thirds had only mild changes. This study demonstrated that individuals with long-standing heartburn treated with antacid therapy have clinical conditions that range from normal findings to potentially severe conditions, including peptic ulcer disease, Barrett's esophagus, and cancer.

A second study, by Corder and coworkers (34), attempted to determine underlying illness in another group of chronic heartburn sufferers. Significant symptoms of more than 3-months' duration that occurred at least once per month for the previous 12 months were required for inclusion. Those who had not consulted their primary care provider for this problem (n = 143) underwent upper endoscopy. Of those individuals who reported symptoms at least once weekly, 68% reported that their symptoms were relieved by antacids (6% were taking H2RAs). Endoscopy revealed that 32% had macroscopic appearances of esophagitis but most were of mild grade. Six patients (4%) had evidence of Barrett's esophagus. Three patients (2%) had mild strictures.

Two additional studies were performed in individuals with less severe disease. To understand better the relationship between objective findings and dyspeptic symptoms, endoscopy was performed in almost the entire population of one small town in Norway (35). Endoscopic abnormalities were identified in 35% of subjects with dyspepsia compared with 38% of those without symptoms. No cases of cancer were discovered.

Simon and coworkers (36) performed endoscopy on individuals enrolled in a trial of OTC famotidine, antacids, and placebo (n =562). At baseline endoscopy, 40% of patients had esophagitis of grade II or above. Peptic ulcer disease was seen in an additional 6%. No occult cancers were detected, most of the abnormal mucosal lesions healed during self-directed treatment, and no complications were encountered (however, the follow-up period was brief).

These findings suggest that for a patient with mild or infrequent symptoms, a medical evaluation is unlikely to reveal underlying pathology that requires intervention. However, patients with long-standing dyspepsia symptoms could benefit from a complete medical consultation and diagnostic work-up.

Failure To Receive Reassurance from Diagnosis Work-Up

A notable criticism of nonprescription therapy (or any treatment strategy without previous diagnostic testing) is the inability to identify an underlying cause of the symptoms. Critics have pointed out that decision-analysis models of dyspepsia management do not include the value of reassurance and satisfaction that can be provided by diagnostic studies (37). Responding to this criticism, Hirth and coworkers (38) used a willingness-to-pay methodology to derive empirically the desire of patients with acid-related symptoms and their physicians to establish a diagnosis. Although almost all of the patients and physicians expressed an interest in knowing their diagnosis, neither group was willing to pay more than $50 for the information (38).

There are conflicting data as to whether patients with normal endoscopic findings are more reassured compared with individuals who are given a cause for their symptoms. Morris and coworkers (39) compared levels of satisfaction and anxiety in dyspepsia patients who had normal endoscopic findings with individuals diagnosed with peptic ulcer disease. Patients with a normal endoscopy reported significant worsening of symptoms over time, greater dissatisfaction with care, and greater anxiety scores. This likely reflects a continued uncertainty in the patient's mind about the diagnosis. These findings suggest that a normal examination may not always provide reassurance and, in certain instances, may make matters worse. In contrast, Bytzer and coworkers (40) found that there was a reduction in physician visits and drug costs in patients who underwent early endoscopy compared with those who underwent empirical therapy. This indirectly implies that early endoscopy reassures patients as to the accuracy of the diagnosis.

Value of Access to Better Therapy

The benefits of a medical consultation include diagnostic and treatment options that may be superior to nonprescription therapy. For individuals who are not completely satisfied with the duration, frequency, and severity of their symptoms, a comprehensive work-up may lead to interventions that improve clinical outcomes. (*See* Chapters 2–6 and 9 for a more detailed discussion of other treatment options).

Conclusions

Dyspepsia is a common symptom associated with varying degrees of morbidity. Due to insufficient pathophysiology and clinical data, an optimal management strategy has not been established. There are clear advantages to permitting self-diagnosis and treatment; however, there are risks associated with the autonomy that comes with self-care. It is unlikely that an accurate risk-benefit calculation for individual patients will ever become available.

Given the available evidence, it seems that the option for self-care is an appropriate one on social, clinical, and economic grounds. Such a choice grants individuals an increased responsibility for their health care decisions. The nonprescription agents seem to be safe and effective. If a person is satisfied with the outcome produced by taking a nonprescription agent, the incremental clinical benefit provided by a medical consultation will be limited. The concern that effective agents mask serious disease is small but real; however, a recommendation that all dyspepsia patients seek professional advice does not seem to be justified. For individuals with long-standing severe heartburn or suspected peptic ulcer disease, a medical consultation may provide important interventions that could improve long-term outcomes. The assessment of the benefits and risks of medical evaluation will need to be reassessed when even more effective therapies (e.g., proton-pump inhibitors) are approved for OTC use.

Key Points

- Although the prevalence of dyspepsia ranges from 13% to 40%, most people with this disorder do not consult a physician for medical care to relieve their symptoms.

- More than 75% of those with dyspepsia use nonprescription drug therapy to relieve their symptoms, making OTC therapy the most common treatment for this group.

- Economic factors have fueled a recent trend to make prescription drugs available as OTC treatments. Costs of pharmaceuticals have shifted from the health payer to the patient, which results in cost savings in managed care settings.

- According to a recent survey, physicians are unlikely to recommend that patients switch from prescription to nonprescription agents.

- Nonprescription options for the treatment of dyspepsia are numerous, with antacids and H2RAs being the most commonly used agents.

- With the introduction of OTC H2RAs, there were expectations of greater symptom relief and fewer office visits; however, these results have not been studied adequately.

- The benefits of nonprescription therapy should be weighed against any possible risks, such as missed diagnoses and failure to receive access to potentially better (e.g., prescription) therapy.

REFERENCES

1. **Jones RH, Lydeard SE.** Prevalence of symptoms of dyspepsia in the community. *BMJ.* 1989;298:30–3.

2. **Drossman DA, Li Z, Andruzzi E.** U.S. Householder Survey of Functional Gastrointestinal Disorders: prevalence, sociodemography, and health impact. *Dig Dis Sci.* 1993;38:1569–80.

3. **Locke GR III.** Prevalence, incidence, and natural history of dyspepsia and functional dyspepsia. *Baillieres Clin Gastroenterol.* 1998;12:435–42.

4. **Johnsen R, Bernersen B, Straume B, et al.** Prevalences of endoscopic and histological findings in subjects with and without dyspepsia. *BMJ.* 1991;302:749–52.

5. **Heikkinen M, Pikkarainen P, Takala J, et al.** Etiology of dyspepsia: four hundred unselected consecutive patients in general practice. *Scand J Gastroenterol.* 1995;30:519–23.

6. **Talley NJ, Boyce P, Jones M.** Identification of distinct upper and lower gastrointestinal symptom groupings in an urban population. *Gut.* 1998;42:690–695.

7. **Marsland DW, Wood M, Mayo F.** Content of family practice. Part I: Rank order of diagnoses by frequency. Part II: Diagnosis by disease category and age/sex distribution. *J Fam Pract.* 1976;3:37–68.

8. **Lydeard S, Jones R.** Factors affecting the decision to consult with dyspepsia: comparison of consulters and non-consulters. *J R Coll Gen Pract.* 1989;39:495–8.

9. **Oliveria SA, Christos PJ, Talley NJ, Dannenberg AJ.** Heartburn risk factors, knowledge, and prevention strategies. *Arch Intern Med.* 1999;159:1592–8.

10. **Graham DY, Smith JL, Patterson DJ.** Why do apparently healthy people use antacid tablets? *Am J Gastroenterol.* 1983;78:257–60.

11. **Fillenbaum GG, Horner RD, Hanlon JT, et al.** Factors predicting change in prescription and nonprescription drug use in a community-residing black and white elderly population. *J Clin Epidemiol.* 1996;49:587–93.

12. **Barber N.** Drugs: from prescription only to pharmacy only. *BMJ.* 1993;307:640.

13. **Andersen M, Schou JS.** Are H$_2$-receptor antagonists safe over-the-counter drugs? *BMJ.* 1994;309:493–4.

14. **Gurwitz JH, McLaughlin TJ, Fish LS.** The effect of an Rx-to-OTC switch on medication prescribing patterns and utilization of physician services: the case of vaginal antifungal products. *Health Serv Res.* 1995;30:672–85.

15. **Porter J.** Increasing the use of nonprescription drugs in a group-model HMO. *Am J Health-System Pharmacy.* 1998;55:1357–8.

16. **Bradley CP, Riaz A, Tobias RS, et al.** Patient attitudes to over-the-counter drugs and possible professional responses to self-medication. *Fam Pract.* 1998;15:44–50.

17. **Erwin J, Britten N, Jones R.** General practitioner's views on the over-the-counter availability of H$_2$-receptor antagonists. *Br J Gen Pract.* 1997;47:99–102.

18. **Editor.** Over-the-counter drugs. *Lancet.* 1994;343:1374–5.

19. **Sena MM, Stoddard ML, Pashko S.** Use of nonantacid anti-ulcer agents in the treatment of heartburn and dyspepsia. *Clin Ther.* 1994;16:103–9.

20. **Severens JL, Laheij RJ, Jansen JB, et al.** Estimating the cost of lost productivity in dyspepsia. *Aliment Pharmacol Ther.* 1998;12:919–23.

21. **Oster G, Huse DM, Delea TE, et al.** The risks and benefits of an Rx-to-OTC switch: the case of over-the-counter H$_2$-blockers. *Med Care.* 1990;28:834–52.

22. **Kalish SC, Bohn RL, Avorn J.** Policy analysis of the conversion of H$_2$-receptor antagonists to over-the-counter use. *Med Care.* 1997;35:32–48.

23. **Wagner PJ, Phillips W, Radford M, Hornsby JL.** Frequent use of medical services: patient reports of intentions to seek care. *Arch Fam Med.* 1995;4:594–9.

24. **Galmiche JP, Letessier E, Scarpignato C.** Fortnightly review: treatment of gastro-oesophageal reflux disease in adults. *BMJ.* 1998;316:1720–3.

25. **Blair DI, Kaplan B, Spiegler J.** Patient characteristics and lifestyle recommendations in the treatment of gastroesophageal reflux disease. *J Fam Pract.* 1997;44:266–72.

26. **Holtmann G, Hotz J, Mayr G, et al.** A double-blind randomized trial on the effects of a herbal preparation in patients with functional dyspepsia. *Gastroenterology.* 1999;116:A65.

27. **Nyren O, Adami H-O, Bates S.** Absence of therapeutic benefit from antacids or cimetidine in nonulcer dyspepsia. *N Engl J Med.* 1986;314:339–43.

28. **Goves J, Oldring JK, Kerr D, et al.** First-line treatment with omeprazole provides an effective and superior alternative strategy in the management of dyspepsia compared to antacid/alginate liquid: a multicentre study in general practice. *Aliment Pharmacol Ther.* 1998;12:147–57.

29. **Graham DY, Patterson DJ.** Double-blind comparison of liquid antacid and placebo in the treatment of reflux esophagitis. *Dig Dis Sci.* 1983;28:559–63.

30. **Goodson JD, Richter JM, Lane RS, et al.** Empirical antacids and reassurance for acute dyspepsia. *J Gen Intern Med.* 1986;1:90–3.

31. **Simon TJ, Gardner AH, Stauffer LA.** Self-directed treatment of intermittent heartburn: a randomized, multicenter, double-blind, placebo-controlled evaluation of famotidine, 5, 10, 20 mg, and antacid. *Gastroenterology.* 1994;106:A181.

32. **Shaw MJ, Kane RL, Fendrick AM.** The impact of over-the-counter H$_2$-receptor antagonists: great expectations unfulfilled. *Gastroenterology.* 1998;114:A41.

33. **Robinson M, Earnest D, Rodriquez-Stanley S, et al.** Heartburn requiring frequent antacid use may indicate significant illness. *Arch Intern Med.* 1998;158: 2373–6.

34. **Corder AP, Jones RH, Sadler GH, et al.** Heartburn, oesophagitis, and Barrett's oesophagus in self-medicating patients in general practice. *Br J Clin Pract.* 1996; 50:245–8.

35. **Bernersen B, Johnsen R, Straume B, Burhol PG.** Erosive prepyloric changes in dyspeptics and nondyspeptics in a defined population: the Sorreisa Gastrointestinal Disorder Study. *Scand J Gastroenterol.* 1992;27:233–7.

36. **Simon TJ, Berlin RG, Gardner AH.** Self-directed treatment of intermittent heartburn: a randomized, multicenter, double-blind, placebo-controlled evaluation of antacid and low doses of an H_2-receptor antagonist (famotidine). *Am J Ther.* 1995; 2:304–13.

37. **Tebaldi M, Heading RC.** Clinical economics review: functional (nonulcer) dyspepsia. *Aliment Pharmacol Ther.* 1998;12:11–9.

38. **Hirth RA, Bloom BS, Chernew ME, Fendrick AM.** Willingness to pay for diagnostic certainty: a comparison among patients, physicians, and managers. *J Gen Intern Med.* 1999;14:193–5.

39. **Morris C, Chapman R, Mayou R.** The outcome of unexplained dyspepsia: a questionnaire follow-up study of patients after endoscopy. *J Psychosom Res.* 1992; 36:751–7.

40. **Bytzer P, Moller-Hansen J, deMuckadell OBS.** Empirical H_2-blocker therapy or prompt endoscopy in management of dyspepsia. *Lancet.* 1994;343:811–6.

9

■ ■ ■

Competing Management Strategies for Dyspepsia: Results of Economic Analyses

Joshua J. Ofman, MD, MSHS

Introduction

This chapter is devoted to a review and critical appraisal of the decision-analysis and economic models that address the management of dyspepsia. It presents the debate over competing management strategies and discusses the various data sources that may contribute to the "evidence" available to decision makers. A discussion of the basis for using economic models follows, providing a framework for critical appraisal of the published decision models for dyspepsia management. How these models add to the "evidence" and how they may affect optimal management strategies for dyspepsia also is discussed. The objectives of this chapter are 1) to explore what dyspepsia research has been done using decision-analysis modeling, 2) to appraise these findings critically using the standard methods of critical appraisal as defined by the Evidence-Based Medicine Working Group (1), and 3) to determine how these findings may determine the "best practices" or the optimal management strategy for dyspepsia patients.

Background

In the past decade, managed care and economic pressures have forced de-

135

cision makers to reevaluate the management of prevalent, costly conditions and to focus on the "efficient" use of medical resources. Concurrently, the discovery of *Helicobacter pylori* as the cause of peptic ulcer disease (PUD) has forced a review of dyspepsia management. The economic issues of dyspepsia management center around three predominant management strategies: empirical antisecretory therapy, initial endoscopy, and most recently testing for and treating *H. pylori* infection.

The optimal management strategy for dyspepsia has been debated since 1985. Kahn and Greenfield (2) performed the first critical evaluation of the published evidence on the "efficacy" of endoscopy in the management of dyspepsia. In proposing guidelines for management, they recommended empirical antisecretory therapy with endoscopy for nonresponders. Their conclusion was based on a lack of evidence that proved a short delay in diagnosis (due to a 4- to 8-week course of empirical therapy) resulted in adverse health outcomes (2). However, debate exists as to the role and timing of endoscopy in the management of dyspepsia (3–12). Because dyspepsia may be caused by PUD, nonulcer dyspepsia (NUD), esophagitis, or gastric cancer, early endoscopy has been advocated to establish a prompt diagnosis and to detect cancer (13–17). In countries with "open access" endoscopy, in which primary care providers may schedule patients for the procedure, this can be accomplished without great expense. In the United States, where subspecialty referral is required and the costs of endoscopy are high, empirical therapy has been advocated, with endoscopy reserved for nonresponders (18).

The lack of consensus about endoscopy's role in dyspepsia management is illustrated by recent studies examining the appropriateness and necessity of endoscopy (19,20). Using RAND/UCLA appropriateness and necessity criteria, which were developed in conjunction with a Swiss expert panel and applied to Swiss ambulatory patients, dyspepsia accounted for 75% of physician visits for upper gastrointestinal complaints. Of the 49% of endoscopies performed for inappropriate indications, 84% were in patients referred for dyspepsia. Moreover, 12% of cases did not have endoscopy performed for "necessary" indications, and dyspepsia was the second most common indication in this group.

The revolution in ulcer therapy that resulted from our recent understanding of the role of *H. pylori* has further confounded the issue and forced a reevaluation of current dyspepsia management strategies. Although consensus has been reached about the role of anti-*H. pylori* therapy in PUD (21), the role of anti-*H. pylori* therapy in NUD remains uncertain for two reasons. First, the epidemiologic evidence of an association between *H. pylori* gastritis and NUD is equivocal (22–24). Second, antibiotic treatment has failed to improve dyspeptic symptoms consistently (25), although serious methodologic problems exist with most randomized placebo-controlled trials addressing this question. Thus, considerable controversy exists over the costs and benefits of noninvasive *H. pylori* testing in patients with dyspepsia (12,26) and whether initial endoscopy or initial anti-*H. pylori* therapy is the optimal management in infected patients (27–29).

The Sources of "Evidence" About Dyspepsia Management

In the climate of constrained health care resources, there is an effort to develop systematic strategies for care that maximize the efficient use of medical resources. How might such strategies be developed and tested? Evidence-based methods for defining "best practices" may rely on several sources of data, with the hope that this evidence-based approach results in the most rational and cost-effective management strategy for improving the health outcomes for dyspepsia patients. The major sources of data include randomized controlled trials (RCTs), effectiveness studies, and decision-analysis models.

Although RCTs represent a time-honored method for evaluating treatment regimens, their results are often difficult to translate into practice for several reasons, including 1) RCTs are often limited by their inability to be generalized to managed care and other settings, 2) RCTs most often compare therapies as opposed to management strategies, and 3) RCT quality can be diminished by methodologic factors such as improper randomization and blinding (30,31).

Effectiveness studies are another source of "evidence" that decision makers can use to determine "best practices." Effectiveness research concerns the results achieved in the actual practice of medical care with typical patients and providers, as opposed to the efficacy of care, which is assessed by the benefits achieved under ideal conditions (32). Although the results of such evaluations may reveal how management strategies or therapies perform in the real world, effectiveness studies—no matter how rigorous—also may suffer from several limitations because 1) they are costly and difficult to implement, 2) randomizing patients is often impossible (thus, the unit of randomization is often the practice setting or the provider), and 3) blinding is rarely feasible. Similar limitations exist for observational studies.

Because the elements of disease-management strategies are rarely evaluated in clinical trials, estimation of the health benefits and costs of management strategies may require modeling. Decision-analysis models can be used to resolve issues of resource allocation and policy decision, but they also may be used to help define "best practices."

The Basis for Using Decision-Analysis Models for Decision Making

Decision analysis is a quantitative method used to compare clinical and economic consequences of alternative management strategies under conditions of uncertainty. Decision models should reflect clinical practice strategies, include an exhaustive set of alternatives for comparison, and be evidence based. Thus, model-probability estimates often are based on the results of RCTs and systematic reviews of the published literature, information derived from administrative databases, and expert opinion. One rationale for modeling clinical decisions using decision analysis may be to explore the effect of uncertainty in model estimates using a process known as sensitivity analysis. This enables the model to test the robustness of each assumption to determine to what extent varying each estimate over a range of uncertainty affects the results of the simulation. Thus, models often indicate which critical variables affect the decision, rather than prescriptively determining the optimal strategy. Particularly, in the absence of large-sale clinical trials or effectiveness studies, decision analysis is a valuable method for exploring the differences in the economic and clinical outcomes of competing strategies for care.

There are several types of economic analyses. *Cost-benefit* analysis presents the cost and outcomes (benefits) in monetary terms and often reports whether a strategy is worth implementing. *Cost-minimization* analysis assumes that outcomes are equivalent and calculates the relative costs of competing strategies. *Cost-effectiveness* analysis presents costs in monetary terms and outcomes in some other unit (e.g., life-years saved, disability-days prevented). *Cost-utility* analysis refers to a cost-effectiveness analysis in which the measure of effectiveness has considered "utilities," such as patient preferences or health-related quality of life so that the measure of effectiveness is quality-adjusted life-years (QALYs). Both cost-effectiveness and cost-utility analyses show how scarce resources may be allocated by computing the relative efficiency of competing strategies. The incremental cost-effectiveness ratio (ICER) defines the amount that must be paid for additional health units using one strategy compared with that of its alternative.

Critical Appraisal of Economic Analyses

The Evidence-Based Medicine Working Group has proposed methods for evaluating the validity and utility of economic analyses (1,33). The critical appraisal of articles assessing the economic effect of health interventions is outlined in Table 9.1. Because economic analyses are generally intended to compare interventions with respect to their resource use and their expected outcomes, they are most useful in helping with allocation decisions rather than dictating them.

The first step in appraising an economic model is to determine whether the results of the analysis are valid—i.e., Did the analysis delineate the strategy that is most efficient or that provides the greatest benefit per unit

Table 9.1   Users' Guide for Economic Analysis of Clinical Practice

Are the Results Valid?

• Did the analysis provide a full economic comparison of health care strategies?

• Were the costs and outcomes properly measured and valued?

• Was appropriate allowance made for uncertainty in the analysis?

• Were estimates of costs and outcomes related to the baseline risk in the treatment population?

What Were the Results?

• What were the incremental costs and outcomes of each strategy?

• Did incremental costs and outcomes differ among subgroups?

• How much did the allowance for uncertainty change the results?

Will the Results Help Me Care for My Patients?

• Are the treatment benefits worth the harms and risks?

• Should my patients expect similar health outcomes?

• Should I expect similar costs?

Republished with permission from Drummond MF, Richardson WS, O'Brien BJ, et al. Users' guides to the medical literature. XIII. How to use an article on economic analysis of clinical practice. A. Are the results of the study valid? Evidence-Based Medicine Working Group. *JAMA*. 1997;277:1552–7.

of resource consumption? The second step is the critiquing the results—i.e., Were the incremental costs and benefits of competing strategies reported? The ICER is most important because it describes how much added health the intervention buys relative to the competing intervention. Although most guidelines on economic analyses suggest that QALYs are the most appropriate unit for cost-effectiveness analysis (34), in many instances (e.g., dyspepsia), the effect on life expectancy is difficult to estimate, as is the effect of interventions on quality of life. A thorough economic analysis also should allow for uncertainty in its estimates and should use sensitivity analysis to test how changing the model estimates might affect the results of the analysis. If the model results are insensitive to changes in key variables, then the model is considered robust. If the model is affected by changes in key variables (within expected ranges of uncertainty based on the medical literature), then the results of the model may not be applicable to the general population.

Finally, you must determine whether the results of the analysis apply to "your" patient population. This includes an appraisal of whether the costs and outcomes demonstrated in the analysis are similar to those in your practice, and this is determined in part by whether the estimates for intervention effects were taken from RCTs (i.e., controlled settings) or "effectiveness" studies (i.e., "real world" studies). Most important, however, is a determination of whether the intervention benefits are worth the harms and costs. If an intervention is both more effective and less costly, then the choice is simple. However, if the intervention is more effective and more costly, then one must weigh the added resources required to achieve additional health benefits against alternative allocation opportunities. This is when using ICERs may be helpful. For example, the ICER for using misoprostol for nonsteroidal anti-inflammatory prophylaxis in rheumatoid arthritis patients is $94,766 per year of life saved; in contrast, the ICER for newborn hepatitis B vaccination is $36,832 per year of life saved. In this situation, a decision maker may decide that the hepatitis vaccine is the preferable investment because it buys more years of life for fewer dollars.

In my review of the economic analyses in dyspepsia management below, I refer to the aforementioned critical appraisal methods. Although a complete appraisal of each analysis is beyond the scope of this chapter, I have attempted to synthesize the findings and to identify where the weight of the evidence lies.

Decision Models in Dyspepsia

Several decision-analysis economic models of dyspepsia management strategies have been published. The rationale has been that there are few prospective, comparative, clinical data about the relative effectiveness of competing strategies. The objective of the models is to help define the most cost-effective management strategy in the absence of perfect information about how each strategy performs in the real world. There are four inherent difficulties that deserve mention in developing and evaluating dyspepsia decision models.

1. **Definition of dyspepsia:** Until recently, there has been a lack of consensus about the definition of dyspepsia. Some definitions have included "reflux-like" dyspepsia, whereas others have not. The recent American Gastroenterological Association guidelines have included the following definition of dyspepsia: pain or discomfort centered in the epigastrium (35). The variable definition of dyspepsia must be considered when evaluating the decision analysis models.

2. **Paucity of prospective comparative data:** Few RCTs have compared management strategies for dyspepsia. One of the first compared empirical antisecretory therapy with initial endoscopy and found that initial endoscopy may result in improved outcomes and decreased costs; however, it did not consider *H. pylori* "test and treat" strategies (36). Other recent data have appeared only in abstract form.

3. **Estimates about the underlying cause of dyspepsia:** Few data exist about the underlying cause in unselected patients presenting with dyspepsia in primary care.

4. **Efficacy of *H. pylori* eradication in NUD:** Treatment trials in NUD are difficult to evaluate due to the high placebo-response rate and methodologic problems with most trials. Although recent RCTs in NUD have resulted in conflicting estimates of the benefit of *H. pylori* eradication in NUD (37,38), previous economic models did not have these data available.

Six economic analyses have addressed the costs or cost effectiveness of competing management strategies in dyspepsia (Table 9.2). Although the first decision analysis detected in our review was performed in 1982 by Read and coworkers (39), this chapter considers only those articles published after 1995, because management strategies and prices for interventions have changed significantly. Economic analyses in which the primary analysis pertained solely to patients with PUD also are excluded from this chapter.

Analysis of Serologic Screening for *Helicobacter pylori*

Sonnenberg (26) developed a cost-benefit analysis of serologic screening for *H. pylori* in subjects with dyspepsia. A decision model was developed to estimate the costs and benefits of *H. pylori* eradication in dyspepsia. The study population was a hypothetical cohort of patients with dyspeptic symptoms. The main effectiveness data were extracted from previously completed studies (from 1989–92) and included the probability of test results, *H. pylori* cure rate, compliance rate, consequences of *H. pylori* eradication, and benefits of the prevention of gastric cancer and peptic ulcer. Resource and cost data were derived mainly from 1987–95 sources. The main outcomes were the probability of *H. pylori* test results, *H. pylori* cure rate, and consequences of *H. pylori* eradication and gastric cancer prevention. Cost estimates related to complications were derived from estimates reported in the medical literature.

The main probability estimates include a conservative 60% *H. pylori* eradication rate (in clinical practice studies in the community, rates have approached 85%–90%). It was assumed that only 10% of dyspepsia patients would have symptoms resolve with *H. pylori* therapy, that only 10% of patients had underlying PUD, and that 0.12% would have gastric cancer prevented by eradicating *H. pylori*.

Based on monetary benefits from the literature—$7000 for PUD prevention, $5000 for the relief of dyspepsia, and $30,000 for cancer prevention—the net benefit of *H. pylori* testing is $1236. The baseline rates showed that the net benefit per patient was $112. A two-way sensitivity

Table 9.2   Economic Models in Dyspepsia

Authors	Clinical Question	Design	Strategies Compared	Results	Comments
Sonnenberg (26)	Should serologic screening for *H. pylori* be performed in dyspepsia?	Cost-benefit analysis	*H. pylori* screening vs. No screening	Net benefit of *H. pylori* screening was $112 per patient	Screening was beneficial so long as 5%–10% of NUD patients respond to *H. pylori* therapy
Fendrick et al. (4)	What is the optimal management strategy for presumed PUD with unknown *H. pylori* status?	Decision analysis and cost-effectiveness analysis	Two invasive strategies (prompt endoscopy with or without biopsy for *H. pylori*) vs. Three noninvasive strategies (serologic *H. pylori* testing and treatment in infected patients, empirical antisecretory therapy, and empirical antisecretory and antimicrobial therapy)	*H. pylori* "test and treat" strategy and empirical antisecretory and antibiotic therapy were most cost effective ($4835 and $4155 per ulcer cured, respectively)	Invasive strategies were equally cost effective when the cost of endoscopy was less than $500
Silverstein et al. (12)	What is the optimal management strategy for patients with a first episode of dyspepsia?	Decision analysis and cost-minimization analysis	Empirical antisecretory therapy vs. Initial endoscopy	Charges for initial endoscopy and empirical therapy were similar ($2163 and $2123 per patient, respectively)	A subanalysis of *H. pylori* "test and treat" strategy was associated with the lowest charges per case ($2109)
Ebell et al. (41)	What is the optimal management strategy for patients with simple dyspepsia?	Decision analysis and cost-utility analysis	Empirical PPI therapy vs. Empirical *H. pylori* eradication vs. Initial endoscopy vs.	*H. pylori* "test and treat" strategy and empirical *H. pylori* therapy were most cost effective ($1214 and $1198 per QALY, respectively)	The model was sensitive to the cost of UGIR, the cost of *H. pylori* testing, and anti-*H. pylori* therapy

			Initial UGIR vs. *H. pylori* "test and treat" strategy vs. Initial UGIR with *H. pylori* serology for ulcers		
Rubin et al. (40)	What is the optimal management strategy for patients with a first episode of dyspepsia?	Decision analysis and cost-minimization analysis	Initial endoscopy or UGIR vs. Initial antisecretory therapy followed by endoscopy or *H. pylori* serology vs. Initial *H. pylori* serology testing	5-year costs were lowest with initial *H. pylori* serology and initial antisecretory therapy followed by serology on relapse compared with initial endoscopy ($1670 and $1950, respectively)	Compared with *H. pylori* serology, initial endoscopy resulted in an incremental cost of $252 for a month of dyspepsia avoided
Ofman et al. (27)	What is the optimal management strategy for *H. pylori* seropositive simple dyspepsia?	Decision analysis and cost-effectiveness analysis	Initial endoscopy vs. Initial anti-*H. pylori* therapy	Initial anti-*H. pylori* therapy resulted in equivalent outcomes, saving $456 per patient and reducing endoscopy workload by 53%	The cost of endoscopy must be reduced by 96% before the two strategies are equally cost effective

NUD = nonulcer dyspepsia; PPI = proton-pump inhibitor; PUD = peptic ulcer disease; QALY = quality-adjusted life year; UGIR = upper gastrointestinal radiography.

analysis was performed on the prevalence rate of PUD and the cure rate of *H. pylori*. A three-way sensitivity analysis included the benefit of ulcer prevention. Only if the benefit of ulcer prevention dropped below $1000 did testing for *H. pylori* in dyspepsia patients become more costly and less beneficial than not testing. A 10% ulcer prevalence rate in *H. pylori*-positive dyspepsia patients required a benefit of at least $4000 associated with ulcer prevention for testing to be more beneficial than not testing. This benefit rose to $6000 with a cure rate of only 60%.

Sonnenberg (26) concluded that, so long as no unequivocal evidence exists that NUD responds to *H. pylori* eradication, treating all *H. pylori*-positive dyspepsia patients cannot be recommended; furthermore, antibiotic therapy should be reserved for patients with proven ulcer or for patients with NUD for whom other measures have failed. However, the analysis reported that so long as 5% to 10% of NUD patients respond to *H. pylori* therapy, then *H. pylori* testing was the most cost-beneficial option, regardless of ulcer prevalence and the benefit associated with ulcer prevention.

There are several limitations to this analysis. The definition of dyspepsia was not stated, so the population to which the analysis applies was not specified. The strength of the analysis depended on the estimates of benefit (dollars saved) by preventing certain outcomes, and the sources and ability of these costs to be generalized remains unclear and may not have been derived from optimal sources. Furthermore, the search to compile the probability estimates was not performed systematically, and there was no measure of the validity of the data sources. Thus, some estimates and ranges of values tested in sensitivity analysis may have been biased.

Analysis Comparing Invasive Testing with Noninvasive Testing in Patients with Suspected Peptic Ulcer Disease

Fendrick and coworkers (4) compared two invasive strategies (prompt endoscopy with or without biopsy for *H. pylori*) with three noninvasive strategies (serologic *H. pylori* testing and treatment in infected patients, empirical antisecretory therapy, and empirical antisecretory and antimicrobial therapy) in the initial management of patients with presumed PUD and unknown *H. pylori* status. Decision analysis was used to model the costs and outcomes of a hypothetical cohort of patients with suspected PUD. The outcome measure was cost per ulcer cured after 1 year.

Literature review was used to derive probability estimates for the model. Important probability estimates included that 20% of patients had underlying active ulcer disease (range 5%–30%). Additionally, the following assumptions were made:

- *H. pylori* was seen more frequently when an ulcer caused the symptoms (95%, range 75%–95%) than when it did not (50%, range 20%–60%).

- The ulcer recurrence rate was higher with *H. pylori* infection (2.7% per 100 patient-months, range 2.0%–6.6%) than without infection (0.6% per 100 patient-months, range 0.1%–2.0%).

- There was a 70% ulcer healing rate after antisecretory therapy (range 50%–90%).

- There was an 80% *H. pylori* eradication rate after antibiotic course (includes compliance) (range 50%–90%).

- The sensitivity and specificity of *H. pylori* serologic testing was 95% (range 50%–100%).

Direct health-service costs were based on actual payments for ambulatory services, inpatient care, and physicians by private third-party payers. Direct costs of pharmaceutical agents were estimated from actual payments made by patients at seven retail pharmacies in three eastern U.S. states.

The estimated benefits and costs were combined using average cost per ulcer cured. No incremental analysis was performed because each strategy was assumed to be equally effective at the conclusion of follow-up. The estimated average treatment costs per ulcer cured by each strategy were as follows:

Strategy 1. Endoscopy and biopsy for *H. Pylori* infection = $8045

Strategy 2. Endoscopy only = $6984

Strategy 3. Serologic test for *H. Pylori* infection = $4541

Strategy 4. Empirical antisecretory therapy = $4835

Strategy 5. Empirical antisecretory and antibiotic therapy = $4155

The analysis revealed that the cost-effectiveness advantage of the noninvasive approaches (strategies 3–5) relative to the immediate endoscopy approaches (strategies 1 and 2) was sensitive to two variables: 1) the cost of endoscopy (endoscopy costs must decrease to less than $500 for an equivalent cost-effectiveness ratio to result), and 2) the probability of recurrent symptoms in patients with NUD (as the annual recurrent symptom rate approached 80%, cost per patient treated of the noninvasive strategies approached that of the immediate invasive diagnostic strategies). Compared with initial serologic testing (strategy 3), the cost-effectiveness advantage of the combined empirical regimen (strategy 5) was sensitive to the cost of the serologic test for *H. pylori* (if the cost of the test were to decrease to $12, an equivalent cost-effectiveness ratio would result).

The results of this analysis suggest that a "test and treat" strategy (serologic testing for *H. pylori* followed by antibiotic therapy in positive patients) may be more cost effective than immediate endoscopy. There are, however, certain limitations to this analysis. In particular, it is unclear whether a systematic review (which limits bias) was performed. This would be necessary to support the validity and relevance of 1) the primary studies that determined which clinical probabilities were used in the decision analysis, and 2) the method of combining the results of the studies. Other concerns about the ability of the costs and probabilities to be generalized were addressed with a comprehensive sensitivity analysis. The study did not consider complications of procedures or side effects related to antibiotic therapy. Additionally, only average, not incremental, cost-effectiveness ratios were reported and used to determine the relative cost effectiveness of competing strategies.

Analyses Comparing Initial Management Strategies in Patients with a First Episode of Dyspepsia

Another decision analysis was performed by Rubin and coworkers (40) who compared initial endoscopy or radiography, initial antisecretory therapy followed by endoscopy or *H. pylori* serology, and initial *H. pylori* serology testing. The primary outcome measure was time spent with symptoms over a 5-year period, and the analysis included direct and indirect costs. Four underlying conditions were considered: PUD, gastroesophageal reflux disease (GERD), functional dyspepsia, and gastric cancer. Probability estimates were derived from the integration of expert opinion and data from published literature. Cost estimates were derived from Medicare reimbursement and average wholesale prices. There was no source for the estimation of indirect costs.

Key model estimates used in the base-case analysis included a 31% rate of underlying GERD in patients with dyspepsia, a 3% rate of early gastric cancer, a 50% *H. pylori* point-prevalence rate, estimates of the annual incidence of bleeding ulcers, an 84% *H. pylori* eradication rate, and a 98.5% sensitivity rate of endoscopy's ability to diagnose early gastric cancer. Indirect cost estimates of lost productivity included 8 hours for each dyspepsia episode, 8 hours for endoscopy, and 2 hours for physician visits. The minimum hourly wage in the United States was used to calculate indirect costs associated with lost productivity.

The five-year costs per patient for each strategy are displayed in Table 9.3. Initial *H. pylori* serology was pronounced to be the most cost-effective strategy, and the results were robust to changing the variable estimates in sensitivity analysis. Although initial endoscopy resulted in 17% higher costs, 36% less time was spent with symptoms and more cancers were diagnosed early. The authors assumed, however, that one-time endoscopy was 98% to 100% accurate in diagnosing early gastric cancer based on a study reporting the results of serial endoscopy with biopsy of gastric ulcers. It is difficult to extrapolate the results of this study to one-time endoscopy of dyspepsia patients without ulcers, and the authors did not report a complete sensitivity analysis around this estimate. The incremental costs of avoiding a month with active dyspepsia compared with initial serology testing were $252 for initial endoscopy and $181 for UGI barium studies per month of active dyspepsia avoided.

Table 9.3   Results from a Decision Analysis

Strategy	5-Year Cost per Patient ($)	Active Dyspepsia Time per Patient Treated (months)	Cancers Diagnosed Early (%)
Endoscopy	1950	2.0	98
Upper gastrointestinal series	1770	2.5	96
Serology	1670	3.1	0
Empirical antisecretory therapy, serology on relapse	1670	4.2	0
Empirical antisecretory therapy and endoscopy on relapse	1750	3.2	0

Republished with permission from Rubin RJ, Cascade EF, Barker RC, et al. Management of dyspepsia: a decision-analysis model. *Am J Manag Care*. 1998;2:647–55.

Another limitation of this analysis is that the authors may not have performed a systematic review to support the validity and relevance of the primary studies that yielded the clinical probabilities used in their decision analysis. It is equally unclear how they derived the methodology for combining the study results with expert opinion. Concerns about the ability of the costs and probabilities to be generalized were addressed with a comprehensive sensitivity analysis. The study did not consider complications of procedures or side effects related to antibiotic therapy. However, the model did attempt to incorporate the incidence of bleeding ulcers and the ability to detect early gastric cancer, estimates for which few data exist. Additionally, it is unclear from what sources the lost productivity data were derived. Although formal cost-effectiveness ratios are not presented, the authors calculated incremental costs for preventing a month of dyspepsia relative to the least costly strategy.

Silverstein and coworkers (12) compared initial management strategies for all patients presenting with a first episode of dyspepsia, including patients with reflux-like symptoms. The two outcome measures were medical charges over 1 year and life expectancy. Decision analysis was used to model two competing strategies in patients with dyspepsia: empirical therapy with an H_2-receptor antagonist and initial upper endoscopy. Four diagnoses were considered in the model: peptic ulcer, gastric cancer, reflux, and functional dyspepsia. Two *H. pylori* strategies also were analyzed. In the first, a positive result would be followed by endoscopy and subsequent treatment based on endoscopic findings. In the second, a positive result would be followed by eradication therapy, with endoscopy reserved for recurrent symptoms. The model considered a 1-year time horizon.

Probability estimates for the model were derived from a review of the medical literature and used a declining exponential approximation of life expectancy (DEALE) to estimate a 0.33 hazard rate per year of gastric cancer. The assumption was made that a 2-month delay in diagnosis would increase this hazard rate by 10% per year. Several assumptions were made about test characteristics for endoscopy in several underlying conditions, but it is unclear from what sources these estimates were derived. Expert opinion was used to supplement literature review to estimate rates of early and late failure of medical therapy. The authors accounted for only direct medical charges—drug charges were taken from a survey of local pharmacies, and other charges were derived from expert opinion and the medical literature.

The analysis found that deciding between initial endoscopy and empiric antisecretory therapy was essentially a "toss-up." Charges were $2163 for initial endoscopy compared with $2123 for empirical therapy. For the *H. pylori* testing strategies, if a positive test was followed by endoscopy, the cost was $2233; if a positive test was followed by eradication therapy, the cost was $2109. This model was highly sensitive to the costs of endoscopy and medical therapy and to the number of recurrent dyspepsia episodes. This is largely because it incorporated lower endoscopy costs and higher probabilities of both failure of therapy and recurrent symptoms than in the aforementioned Fendrick model (4). The difference in life expectancy between strategies was approximately 3 days in a cohort of dyspepsia patients who were 55 years of age.

This study is limited by the fact that it reports only total medical charges, rather than a measure of cost effectiveness. Moreover, it is unclear whether the cost and probability estimates were obtained using a systematic method that minimizes bias. This is particularly important for the estimates of gastric cancer risk, outcomes, and the test characteristics of endoscopy. Additionally, the method used to obtain and incorporate expert opinion is not stated explicitly and the study did not consider complications of procedures or side effects related to antibiotic therapy. This study demonstrates that life expectancy is not the most relevant outcome measure when comparing management strategies for dyspepsia.

Analysis Comparing Management Strategies in Patients with Simple Dyspepsia

In an effort to incorporate *quality* of life rather than merely *quantity* of life (i.e., life expectancy) into the outcomes of dyspepsia, Ebell and coworkers (41) performed a cost-utility analysis for patients with simple dyspepsia (i.e., those with no signs or symptoms of complications) (Table 9.4). Seven strategies in the primary care setting were compared:

1. Antisecretory therapy for 1 month with omeprazole

2. Empirical *H. pylori* eradication

3. Upper endoscopy as a diagnostic test to identify patients for *H. pylori* eradication

4. Upper gastrointestinal barium study as a diagnostic test

5. *H. pylori* serology, followed by *H. pylori* eradication in patients testing positive

6. Upper endoscopy as an initial diagnostic test, followed by serum titer for *H. pylori* if positive for ulcer

7. Upper gastrointestinal radiography as an initial diagnostic test, followed by serum titer for *H. pylori* if positive for ulcer

Table 9.4   Results of a Cost-Utility Analysis

Strategy	*Symptomatic Ulcer Recurrence Probability (%)*	*Deaths per 100,000 Patients*	*1-Year Cost per Patient ($)*	*Cost per Ulcer Cured ($/cure)*	*Utility (QALY)*	*Cost Utility ($/QALY)*
Empirical *H. pylori* eradication	1.3	2.6	1197	5781	0.9987	1198
H. pylori "test and treat" strategy	1.4	2.8	1213	5891	0.9990	1214
Empirical omeprazole for 1 month	3.5	7.0	1286	1286	0.9991	1288
Initial UGIR and *H. pylori* serology if ulcer present	1.8	3.7	1452	1452	0.9981	1455
Initial UGIR and *H. pylori* eradication if ulcer present	1.7	3.5	1509	1510	0.9981	1512
Initial endoscopy and *H. pylori* eradication if ulcer present	1.5	3.0	2109	2110	0.9982	2114
Initial endoscopy and *H. pylori* serology if ulcer present	1.7	3.4	2125	2126	0.9982	2130

QALY = quality-adjusted life year.
Republished with permission from Ebell MH, Warbasse L, Brenner C. Evaluation of the dyspeptic patient: a cost-utility study. *J Fam Pract.* 1997;44:545–55.

Four diagnoses were considered: duodenal ulcer, gastric ulcer, gastric malignancy, and NUD. Dyspepsia was defined by the authors as upper abdominal pain. The time horizon of the model was 1 year.

Probability estimates were derived from a review of the MEDLARS bibliographic database. There were no explicit inclusion or exclusion criteria or quality-assessment methods given for literature retrieval. Key probability estimates incorporated in the model included the probabilities of a dyspepsia patient having a duodenal ulcer (0.14) and of triple therapy being successful in eradicating *H. pylori* at 1 week (0.85). The sensitivity and specificity of a serum immunoglobulin G (IgG) titer for *H. pylori* were 0.90 and 0.95, respectively.

Drug cost estimates were obtained from a survey of five pharmacies. Other costs (e.g., upper endoscopy, office visits, serum IgG for *H. pylori*, upper gastrointestinal radiography, hospitalization for gastrointestinal bleeding, hospitalization for ulcer surgery) were calculated based on the data obtained from five health institutions. The cost per dyspepsia episode for each strategy was estimated from the payer's perspective.

The utility of delaying cancer diagnosis by 6 weeks was 0.7433. The range of the utilities associated with the health states was between 0.4642 and 0.7604. A formula was used to calculate the disutility of events (QALYs lost) based on utilities attributed to health states by the Index of Well-Being (IWB). The disutility (QALYs lost) associated with the health state of delaying diagnosis of cancer for 6 weeks was 0.030. The corresponding value for experiencing upper endoscopy, for example, was 0.001. The total range from the highest utility strategy (antisecretory therapy for 1 month with omeprazole) to the lowest utility strategy (an upper gastrointestinal series) was only 0.001 QALY. The differences in QALYs were considered clinically insignificant.

The secondary measures of benefits were the rates of symptomatic ulcer recurrence and death. Empirical *H. pylori* eradication had the lowest probability of symptomatic ulcer recurrence (1.3% of all dyspepsia patients) and death (2.6 deaths per 100,000 dyspepsia patients). The highest ulcer recurrence and death rates were associated with empirical antisecretory therapy (3.5% and 7, respectively). The side effects of treatments were considered in this analysis.

The highest cost per dyspepsia episode was associated with upper endoscopy ($2125.99). The primary measure of cost-utility was cost per QALY. The most cost-effective strategy was empirical *H. pylori* eradication ($1198 per QALY), followed by *H. pylori* titer with eradication therapy for those who tested positive ($1214 per QALY), and empirical omeprazole ($1288 per QALY). However, empirical antisecretory therapy was shown to be associated with higher morbidity and mortality rates than the other two strategies. One-way sensitivity analysis showed that the model was sensitive to the cost of upper gastrointestinal radiography, *H. pylori* serology, and *H. pylori* eradication.

A limitation of this analysis is that the method for deriving utility estimates was not explained. A systematic approach to combining and/or taking weighted averages for deriving probability estimates also was not clearly stated. Furthermore, the incremental cost-utility ratio was not calculated because the differences in the utilities were not clinically significant.

Summarizing the findings of the above five economic analyses, it seems that *H. pylori* testing is a cost-effective approach when compared with invasive strategies. These results hold true despite varying the model estimates over a wide range of uncertainty. In many cases, the results were sensitive to the costs of endoscopy, which when substantially reduced, may be the most cost-effective initial strategy. Although the economic models support the use of an *H. pylori* "test and treat" approach, scant data can direct optimal management for those who are *H. pylori* seropositive. Most of the economic models previously referenced assumed that seropositive patients should be treated for *H. pylori* rather than investigated to define PUD. Because documented PUD remains the only consensus indication for anti-*H. pylori* therapy (21), European studies have focused on using *H. pylori* serology to identify seropositive patients for endoscopy to reduce the endoscopy workload (28,29,42). Although this strategy makes sense in an "open access" system, it may not be appropriate in the U.S. system in which dyspepsia management has been traditionally based on empirical therapy (18).

Analysis Comparing Initial Endoscopy with Anti-*Helicobacter pylori* Therapy in *Helicobacter pylori*-Seropositive Patients

In an effort to resolve the discordant approaches, a recent decision analysis compared initial endoscopy with initial anti-*H. pylori* therapy in seropositive patients with dyspepsia (27). The model assumed that long-term clinical outcomes were equivalent. The outcome measures were costs and the complications of endoscopy and antibiotic use. A systematic literature review was performed to derive model estimates, and costs were taken form the perspective of a third-party payer. Important probability estimates included an underlying 25% prevalence of PUD in seropositive patents (range 15%–35%), a 45% response rate in NUD patients to anti-*H. pylori* therapy (range 30%–70%) and an 80% *H. pylori* eradication rate (range 60%–95%). Antibiotic and endoscopic complications were considered in this analysis. Costs included Medicare reimbursements for procedures, physician fees, facility fees, and hospitalizations related to cancer and complications. Pharmacy costs were derived from a health maintenance organization's pharmacy cost-accounting system.

The average cost per patient was calculated, and equivalent long-term outcomes were assumed. Initial anti-*H. pylori* therapy cost $820 compared with $1276 for endoscopy, resulting in a savings of $456 per patient treated. Initial anti-*H. pylori* therapy also resulted in a 53% reduction in the endoscopy workload, without compromising clinical outcomes at 1 year. Thus, if patients with uncomplicated dyspepsia are tested for *H. pylori*, then initial anti-*H. pylori* therapy is more cost-effective than initial endoscopy. The cost of endoscopy must be reduced by 96% before the two strategies become equally cost effective. The model was not sensitive to the therapeutic effect of anti-*H. pylori* therapy in NUD patients.

Although this analysis included the costs of endoscopic and antibiotic-related complications, it is limited by a lack of formal pooling methods for deriving probability estimates. Additionally, the authors accounted for direct costs only and incremental cost-effectiveness ratios were not calculated because outcomes were assumed to be equivalent in both strategies.

Thus, contrary to the approach adopted by European studies, this study suggests that the optimal approach for *H. pylori* seropositive patients with dyspepsia should be empirical anti-*H. pylori* therapy. Several studies reported the effect of changing endoscopy costs on the decision to use a "test and treat" strategy compared with initial invasive testing. Although the endoscopy costs used in the analyses vary, the extent to which they must change is the critical factor. Table 9.5 illustrates the varying degrees to which endoscopy costs affect the decision to choose alternative management strategies.

Conclusions

Economic analyses are best used only to inform clinical decision making, rather than to provide "answers" or prescriptive recommendations. The optimal management strategy for patients with dyspepsia will be elucidated when prospective trials define the strategy that results in improved patient outcome at an acceptable investment of resources (considering both direct and indirect costs). The most cost-effective strategy may be one that is more, rather than less, costly so long as decision makers determine that the additional health benefits are worth the additional costs. Thus, focusing on the least costly strategy may not provide practitioners with the optimal management recommendations.

Most of the analyses reviewed in this chapter did not provide a complete evaluation of treatment strategies. These were frequently limited to 1 year of therapy, did not consider important outcomes such as complications and side effects, and did not consider the long-term effect on quality of life. Because most patients with dyspepsia have NUD, it may be assumed that the initial management strategy should not affect long-term outcomes. Thus, elucidating the utilities and benefits of health-related quality of life in NUD patients may be the best way to inform decision making in

Table 9.5   Endoscopy Costs in Analyses Comparing Endoscopy with Competing Strategies

Authors	Base-Case Endoscopy with Biopsy Costs ($)	Base-Case Endoscopy with Biopsy (and Pathology) Costs ($)	Range Tested ($)	Results of Sensitivity Analysis
Fendrick et al. (4)	2102*	—	200–2000	Endoscopy costs must decrease to less than $500 for it to be equally cost effective
Silverstein et al. (12)	585	—	0–1500	If the costs of endoscopy are below $277, then initial endoscopy is the preferred strategy
Ebell et al. (41)	1000*	—	200–1500	—
Rubin et al. (40)	623	712	200–400	At $365, endoscopy is always preferred to UGIR; however, across this range, serology is always preferable to endoscopy
Ofman et al. (27)	713*	1025*	0–110	Endoscopy costs must be reduced by 96% before it is equally cost effective

* Including facility fees.

the long-term, yet it may not affect the decision about what is the optimal initial management strategy. Most analyses conclude that initial noninvasive strategies for dyspepsia management, particularly *H. pylori* "test and treat" strategies, save money by avoiding endoscopy in a subset of patients and by curing ulcers in those with *H. pylori*-associated PUD. Because nonresponders undergo endoscopy in all of the economic models, long-term outcomes among strategies should not be affected. Although several attempts were made to define the consequence of a delayed diagnosis of gastric cancer on life expectancy or cost utility, the effect was clinically insignificant in all cases and the data on which these assumptions rest were not based on relevant, well-designed clinical studies.

Until the results of prospective RCTs performed in several practice settings are completed, the economic analyses reviewed here may be used to guide decisions about the optimal initial management strategy. These analyses suggest that, in patients with uncomplicated dyspepsia, noninvasive strategies (e.g., *H. pylori* "test and treat" strategy) may be the most cost-efficient management options that result in equivalent or improved patient outcomes. If this strategy is adopted, attention must be paid to the population selected (patients with predominant GERD symptoms and/or warning signs of serious organic pathology [e.g., anemia, vomiting, weight loss] must be excluded). Moreover, this strategy includes the use of endoscopy in patents with persistent dyspepsia symptoms despite successful cure of the *H. pylori* infection.

■ ■ ■

Key Points

- Managed care has resulted in an increased need for evaluating the cost effectiveness of diagnostic and management approaches.

- Recent changes in ulcer therapy have contributed to the reevaluation of dyspepsia management strategies (e.g., the appropriateness of anti-*H. pylori* therapy in NUD).

- Economic models evaluating dyspepsia management strategies have been hindered by some difficulties, including 1) a lack of consensus about the definition of dyspepsia, 2) insufficient comparative data, 3) uncertainty about the underlying causes of dyspepsia, and 4) high placebo-response rates in many trials.

- Based on the results of five economic analyses, *H. pylori* testing as the initial strategy is more cost effective than are invasive strategies (e.g., endoscopy with or without biopsy) so long as the patients selected do not have "alarm symptoms" of serious disease or symptoms of predominant GERD.

■ ■ ■

REFERENCES

1. **Drummond MF, Richardson WS, O'Brien BJ, et al.** Users' guides to the medical literature. XIII. How to use an article on economic analysis of clinical practice. A.

Are the results of the study valid? Evidence-Based Medicine Working Group. *JAMA*. 1997;277:1552–7.

2. **Kahn KL, Greenfield S.** The efficacy of endoscopy in the evaluation of dyspepsia: a review of the literature and development of a sound strategy. *J Clin Gastroenterol.* 1986;8:346–58.

3. **Axon AT.** Chronic dyspepsia: Who needs endoscopy? *Gastroenterology.* 1997;112:1376–80.

4. **Fendrick AM, Chernew ME, Hirth RA, Bloom BS.** Alternative management strategies for patients with suspected peptic ulcer disease. *Ann Intern Med.* 1995;123:260–8.

5. **Fennerty MB.** Empirical H_2-blocker therapy or prompt endoscopy in the management of dyspepsia. *Gastrointest Endosc.* 1995;41:529–30.

6. **Rabeneck L.** Managing dyspepsia: Is prompt endoscopy the way to go? *Gastroenterology.* 1995;108:1324–6.

7. **Williams B, Luckas M, Ellingham JH, et al.** Do young patients with dyspepsia need investigation? *Lancet.* 1988;2:1349–51.

8. **Jones R.** When is endoscopy appropriate in dyspepsia? (Editorial). *Am J Gastroenterol.* 1993;88:981–2.

9. **Johnsen R.** Endoscopy: why and when (Editorial). *Scand J Prim Health Care.* 1990;8:187–8.

10. **Malagelada JR.** When and how to investigate the dyspeptic patient. *Scand J Gastroenterol Suppl.* 1991;182:70–4.

11. **Colin-Jones DG.** When should endoscopy (or radiology) be used in dyspepsia and peptic ulcer disease? *Aliment Pharmacol Ther.* 1987;1(Suppl 1):548–55S.

12. **Silverstein MD, Petterson T, Talley NJ.** Initial endoscopy or empirical therapy with or without testing for *Helicobacter pylori* for dyspepsia: a decision analysis. *Gastroenterology.* 1996;110:72–83.

13. **Mansi C, Mela GS, Savarino V, et al.** Open access endoscopy: a large-scale analysis of its use in dyspeptic patients. *J Clin Gastroenterol.* 1993;16:149–54.

14. **Heatley RV.** Open-access upper gastrointestinal endoscopy: visions of the future or the past? *Br J Hosp Med.* 1994;51:366–9.

15. **Hallissey MT, Allum WH, Jewkes AJ, et al.** Early detection of gastric cancer. *BMJ.* 1990;301:513–5.

16. **Nyren O.** Therapeutic trial in dyspepsia: its role in the primary care setting. *Scand J Gastroenterol Suppl.* 1991;182:61–9.

17. **Bytzer P.** Diagnosing dyspepsia: any controversies left? (Editorial). *Gastroenterology.* 1996;110:302–6.

18. **ACP Health and Public Policy Committee.** Endoscopy in the evaluation of dyspepsia. *Ann Intern Med.* 1985;102:266–9.

19. **Froehlich F, Burnand B, Pache I, et al.** Overuse of upper gastrointestinal endoscopy in a country with open-access endoscopy: a prospective study in primary care. *Gastrointest Endoscop.* 1997;45:13–9.

20. **Froehlich F, Pache I, Burnand B, et al.** Underutilization of upper gastrointestinal endoscopy. *Gastroenterology.* 1997;112:690–7.

21. **NIH Consensus Development Panel on *Helicobacter pylori* in Peptic Ulcer Disease.** *Helicobacter pylori* in peptic ulcer disease. *JAMA.* 1994;272:65–9.

22. **Greenberg RE, Bank S.** The prevalence of *Helicobacter pylori* in nonulcer dyspepsia: importance of stratification according to age. *Arch Intern Med.* 1990;150: 2053–5.

23. **Johnsen R, Bernersen B, Straume B, et al.** Prevalences of endoscopic and histological findings in subjects with and without dyspepsia. *BMJ.* 1991;302:749–52.

24. **Talley NJ.** The role of *Helicobacter pylori* in nonulcer dyspepsia: a debate—against. *Gastroenterol Clin North Am.* 1993;22:153–67.

25. **Talley NJ.** A critique of therapeutic trials in *Helicobacter pylori*-positive functional dyspepsia. *Gastroenterology.* 1994;106:1174–83.

26. **Sonnenberg A.** Cost-benefit analysis of testing for *Helicobacter pylori* in dyspeptic subjects. *Am J Gastroenterol.* 1996;91:1773–7.

27. **Ofman JJ, Etchason J, Fullerton S, et al.** Management strategies for *Helicobacter pylori*-seropositive patients with dyspepsia: clinical and economic consequences. *Ann Intern Med.* 1997;126:280–91.

28. **Patel P, Khulusi S, Mendall MA, et al.** Prospective screening of dyspeptic patients by *Helicobacter pylori* serology. *Lancet.* 1995;346:1315–8.

29. **Sobala GM, Crabtree JE, Pentith JA, et al.** Screening dyspepsia by serology to *Helicobacter pylori. Lancet.* 1991;338:94–6.

30. **Jadad AR, Moore RA, Carroll D, et al.** Assessing the quality of reports of randomized clinical trials: Is blinding necessary? *Control Clin Trials.* 1996;17:1–12.

31. **Moher D, Jadad AR, Tugwell P.** Assessing the quality of randomized controlled trials: current issues and future directions. *Int J Technol Assess Health Care.* 1996;12:195–208.

32. **Brook RH, Lohr KN.** Monitoring quality of care in the Medicare program: two proposed systems. *JAMA.* 1987;258:3138–41.

33. **O'Brien BJ, Heyland D, Richardson WS, et al.** Users' guides to the medical literature. XIII. How to use an article on economic analysis of clinical practice. B. What are the results and will they help me in caring for my patients? Evidence-Based Medicine Working Group. *JAMA.* 1997;277:1802–6.

34. **Weinstein MC, Siegel JE, Gold MR, et al.** Recommendations of the Panel on Cost-Effectiveness in Health and Medicine. *JAMA.* 1996;276:1253–8.

35. **American Gastroenterological Association.** Medical position statement: evaluation of dyspepsia. *Gastroenterology.* 1998;114:579–81.

36. **Bytzer P, Hansen JM, Schaffalitzky de Muckadell OB.** Empirical H_2-blocker therapy or prompt endoscopy in management of dyspepsia. *Lancet.* 1994;343: 811–6.

37. **Blum AL, Talley NJ, O'Morain C, et al.** Lack of effect of treating *Helicobacter pylori* infection in patients with nonulcer dyspepsia: Omeprazole plus Clarithromycin and Amoxicillin effect one year after Treatment (OCAY) Study Group. *N Engl J Med.* 1998;339:1875–81.

38. **McColl K, Murray L, el-Omar E, et al.** Symptomatic benefit from eradicating *Helicobacter pylori* infection in patients with nonulcer dyspepsia. *N Engl J Med.* 1998;339:1869–74.

39. **Read L, Pass TM, Komaroff AL.** Diagnosis and treatment of dyspepsia: a cost-effectiveness analysis. *Med Decis Making.* 1982;2:415–38.

40. **Rubin RJ, Cascade EF, Barker RC, et al.** Management of dyspepsia: a decision-analysis model. *Am J Manag Care.* 1998;2:647–55.

41. **Ebell MH, Warbasse L, Brenner C.** Evaluation of the dyspeptic patient: a cost-utility study. *J Fam Pract.* 1997;44:545–55.

42. **Tham TC, Van Dam J.** Prospective screening of dyspeptic patients by *Helicobacter pylori* serology. *Gastrointest Endosc.* 1996;43:532–4.

10

■ ■ ■

Alternative Medical Therapies for Dyspepsia: A Systematic Review of Randomized Trials

Brooks D. Cash, MD

Philip Schoenfeld, MD, MSEd, MSc(Epi)

The opinions and assertions contained herein are the sole opinions of the authors and are not to be construed as being official or reflecting the policy of the U.S. Department of the Navy or the U.S. Department of Defense.

The Office of Alternative Medicine of the National Institutes of Health has formally defined *alternative and complementary medicine* as "a broad domain of healing resources that encompasses all health systems, modalities, and practices, and their accompanying theories and beliefs, other than those intrinsic to the politically dominant health system" (1). With this broad definition, it is not surprising that the range of available alternative medicine therapies ranges from acupuncture to healing touch to behavioral modification to herbal therapy (Table 10.1). Notably, the use of alternative medicine therapies has increased rapidly in the 1990s. In 1997, 42% of U.S. citizens used these therapies and out-of-pocket expenditures exceeded $12 billion (2). Given the rapid increase in the use of alternative medicine therapies, physicians need to understand the indications and complications associated with alternative medicine (3).

The use of alternative medicine is not confined to patients dissatisfied with conventional medicine; 40% of patients who are satisfied with conventional medicine also use alternative medicine therapies, and only 4.4% of all patients disregard conventional medical treatments and rely solely on alternative medicine therapies (4). Thus, most patients use alternative medi-

Table 10.1   Alternative Medicine Headings in MEDLINE

• Acupuncture	• Medicine, Traditional
• Anthroposophy	• Mental Healing
• Biofeedback	• Moxibustion
• Chiropractic	• Music Therapy
• Color Therapy	• Naturopathy
• Diet Fads	• Organotherapy
• Eclecticism	• Radiesthesis
• Electrical Stimulation Therapy	• Reflexotherapy
• Homeopathy	• Relaxation Techniques
• Kinesiology, Applied	• Therapeutic Touch
• Massage	• Tissue Therapy

cine therapies as a supplement. Patients are more likely to use these therapies if they have chronic pain (odds ratio [OR] = 2.0; 95% confidence interval [CI] = 1.1–3.5) and anxiety (OR = 3.1; 95% CI = 1.6–6.0) (4). Based on the chronic discomfort and anxiety associated with functional bowel disorders, it is not surprising that patients with such disorders frequently seek care from alternative medicine practitioners (5).

Although no single treatment has consistently improved nonulcer dyspepsia (NUD) symptoms, multiple interventions have been used, including H_2-receptor antagonists, prokinetic agents, proton-pump inhibitors, antiemetics, anticholinergic agents, and dietary modification (6). Given the limited efficacy of conventional medical treatments for NUD, patients with NUD frequently seek out alternative medicine therapies. However, before alternative medicine therapies can be routinely applied to the treatment of NUD, rigorously designed research must be performed and analyzed to identify the safest and most effective of these therapies.

To our knowledge, no previous systematic review has assessed the effectiveness of alternative medicine therapies in the treatment of NUD. Therefore, we conducted a review of randomized trials that studied the efficacy of herbal medicine, acupuncture, and psychotherapy and hypnotherapy in NUD patients. Due to the limited understanding of these alternative medicine therapies, we also have provided a primer on the indications and complications associated with herbal medicine, the philosophy and practice of traditional Chinese herbal medicine and acupuncture, and a brief review of psychotherapeutic modalities used to treat functional bowel disorders.

Review of Alternative Medicine Therapies

Uses and Adverse Reactions Associated with Herbal Medicine

Popular herbal medicines include St. John's wort, ginseng, gingko, *Echinacea*, and milk thistle (7). An overview of the indications, side effects, drug interactions, and dosing of the most common herbal medicines are provided in Table 10.2. When reviewing Table 10.2, several caveats about commonly used herbal medicines should be considered. Because the production of herbal medicine is not regulated by the Food and Drug Administration, contaminant or variable doses of active ingredients are frequently found in herbal products. Ephedra (ma huang) contains ephedrine and/or pseudoephedrine, the amount of which may vary considerably, leading to multiple complications from excess cholinergic stimulation. Multiple contaminations have been reported with herbal medicines imported from China, including contaminations with lead, mercury, and arsenic (8). Also, aconitine poisoning, anticholinergic overdose, mineralocorticoid excess, *Podophyllin* poisoning, and heavy metal poisoning all have been reported with Chinese herbal therapies due to faulty processing of the preparation, variability of the active ingredients included, or chronic use of preparations containing aconitine or anticholinergics (9). Given these concerns, users of herbal medicine should review labeling to confirm that a specific dose of the active herbal ingredient is present and should seek herbal medicines produced by reputable U.S. manufacturers.

Several additional warnings about the use and misuse of alternative medicine therapies also should be noted. Comfrey (*Symphytum officinale*) is used as a topical gel on minor cuts, which reportedly facilitates healing. It is also sold in oral forms (e.g., teas, tablets) for the treatment of stomach ulcers. However, oral ingestion of comfrey has been associated with hepatitis. Kava kava may have a muscle-relaxant effect and is frequently prescribed as a sedative. If it is mixed with other sedative agents, then significant central nervous system side effects have been reported (8). Finally, gingko, which has been reported to sharpen memory and cognition, is contraindicated for patients taking aspirin or warfarin due to gingko's anticoagulant effect. These caveats may be especially beneficial when your patients ask about the safety of different herbal medications and drug interactions.

Philosophy of Traditional Chinese Herbal Medicine and Acupuncture

Traditional Chinese medicine was derived from Taoism more than 4000 years ago and has the Qi (pronounced "Chee") as its central concept. Qi, which means "vital energy," is thought to be the element that separates life from death (10). Each individual is thought to have a unique supply and distribution of Qi that, in health, flows unobstructed through various chan-

Table 10.2   Overview of Commonly Used Herbal Products

Herb	Indication	Side Effects	Drug Interactions and Contraindications	Dosage
Ginseng	Lack of stamina, need for invigoration, convalescence	Overdose may result in ginseng abuse syndrome (e.g., sleeplessness, hypertonia, edema) and possible estrogenic effects	None known	1–2 g/d (root) administered as comminuted drug infusion, powder, or Galenic preparation
St. John's wort	Anxiety, depressed mood, skin inflammation, blunt injuries, wounds, burns	Fullness or constipation, photosensitivity	None known	Internal: 2–4 g/d as a liquid External: 0.2–1.0 mg/d as a liquid or semi-solid preparation
Gingko	Organic brain dysfunction, claudication, vascular vertigo, vascular tinnitus	Gastrointestinal complaints, allergic skin reactions, muscle spasms, cramps, atonia, adynamia	Potential to interact with antithrombotic therapy	120 mg bid–tid of dried extract orally
Echinacea	Fevers and colds, cough/bronchitis, urinary tract infections, tendency to infection, wounds and burns	Fever, nausea, vomiting	None known; avoid parenteral administration in pregnancy; exercise caution in patients with tuberculosis, AIDS, collagen vascular disorders	Variable depending on species administered
Milk thistle	Dyspepsia, loss of appetite, liver and gall bladder complaints	Mild diarrhea	None known	12–15 g/d as an infusion or tincture
Feverfew	Migraine, arthritis, rheumatic diseases, allergies	Skin hypersensitivity, contact dermatitis	Possibility of interactions with antithrombotic medications; do not use in pregnant or nursing patients	50 mg/d–1.2 g/d for internal or external use
Comfrey	Gastric ulcers, gastritis, blunt injuries	None	Pyrrolizdine alkaloids; do not use in pregnant or nursing patients	Variable depending on species administered; used internally and as an ointment
Ephedra	Cough, bronchitis, asthma	Headache, irritability, motor restlessness, tachycardia, nausea, hypertension, dependence	Cardiac glycosides, guanethidine, MAOIs, oxytocin	300 mg/d as a tea, tincture, or extract
Garlic	Dyspepsia, bloating, arteriosclerosis, colds, fevers, cough, bronchitis, hypercholesterolemia	Hand eczema with prolonged contact, occasional gastrointestinal distress	May interact with antithrombotic medications	4 g/d as fresh garlic; 8 mg/d essential garlic oil
Saw palmetto	Prostatism, irritable bladder	Occasional gastrointestinal complaints	Avoid in pregnancy or nursing	1–2 g/d orally
Peppermint oil	Dyspepsia, liver and gall bladder complaints, loss of appetite, nausea, vomiting, fevers, colds, myalgias	Possible biliary colic due to cholagogic effect	Biliary obstruction, cholecystitis, liver insufficiency, severe GERD	Comminuted herb: 3–6 g/d (5–15 g/d of tincture) Essential oil: 6–12 drops per day; 0.6 mL enteric coated for IBS

GERD = gastroesophageal reflux disease; IBS = irritable bowel syndrome; MAOIs = monoamine-oxidase inhibitors.

nels in the body. Each person's Qi is freely exchanged with the Qi present throughout the environment. When this exchange is blocked or the flow otherwise deranged, physical or mental illness can occur (11). Both traditional Chinese herbal therapy and acupuncture seek to bring the body and mind back into balance with the environment to restore health.

Chinese herbal therapy uses naturally occurring products that have been prepared by a trained "herbalist" as a decoction and individualized to the patient. Over 6000 different medicinal plants are used. Herbalists combine eight to 12 different plants to ensure that the preparation "realigns" the multiple parts of the body that are out of balance. However, only 230 medicinal plants have been subjected to any kind of in-depth pharmacobiologic analysis (9).

Acupuncture also has been used as a therapeutic intervention for more than 4000 years (12,13). As with Chinese herbal medicine, acupuncture is designed to regulate the flow of Qi through the body to correct the disordered "flow" that has caused the disease requiring treatment. Solid needles are inserted 0.5 to 0.8 cm (depending on the location) into the skin and manipulated manually, stimulated electrically, or heated by burning a dried herb (mugwort) over the point or needle. The practitioner inserts needles along 12 well-mapped meridians and channels through which the Qi is thought to flow. Reported complications include bleeding, infection, pneumothorax, and perforated viscus (14).

Psychotherapy and Hypnotherapy

Psychotherapy includes the use of structured and nonstructured interviews between therapists and patients designed to identify and modify patient response to psychosocial stressors. Different psychotherapeutic modalities used to treat functional bowel disorders include insight-oriented psychotherapy, relaxation and stress management training, cognitive-based behavioral therapy, biofeedback, and hypnotherapy (15). The most studied of these modalities is cognitive-behavioral therapy. This form of psychotherapy is designed to teach patients how to identify their maladaptive behavior and manage their responses to stressful life events or situations. The psychotherapy treatment program is frequently given as a "treatment package" that includes a combination of traditional psychotherapy, biofeedback training, relaxation techniques, muscle relaxation techniques, and basic physiologic education about the functions of the gastrointestinal system (16).

Methods

Literature Search

MEDLINE searches of English-language articles from 1970 to 1998 were performed to identify relevant studies. The following medical subject headings (MeSH) terms were used in the searches: dyspepsia, abdominal pain, irritable bowel syndrome (IBS), alternative medicine, acupuncture, herbal therapy, diet, psychotherapy, biofeedback, and hypnotherapy. The bibliographies of all primary studies and of selected review articles were searched manually to identify additional relevant studies. (Note: Due to the paucity of rigorously designed trials in NUD, we included rigorously designed trials of alternative medicine therapies in IBS patients; 42% of patients with NUD also meet diagnostic criteria for IBS, demonstrating a significant overlap between these functional bowel disorders [17].)

Study Selection Criteria

Independent duplicate review of the titles and abstracts of all citations from the MEDLINE searches was performed. All potentially relevant studies identified by either of the reviewers were retrieved. One investigator then independently reviewed the full manuscript of all potentially relevant studies and applied the following selection criteria:

- Randomized trial using a crossover or parallel design
- Population of adult patients with NUD or IBS
- Randomized comparison of alternative medicine therapy with placebo or conventional medical therapy
- Evaluation of gastrointestinal symptoms or generic quality of life

Data Extraction and Analysis

Data extraction was performed on the following:
- Randomization procedures
- Use of placebo
- Blinding of physicians, patients, and outcome adjudicators
- Patient population
- Choice of medications and dosing schedule
- Duration of study
- Assessment of gastrointestinal symptoms or generic quality of life
- Side effects

Data about patient population, study design, study intervention, and outcome measures are provided in Tables 10.3 and 10.4. The wide variation in study design and intervention prevented pooling of data. Therefore, study results are not presented in a statistical summary and are simply described in the "Results" section below.

Table 10.3   Traditional Chinese Herbal Medicine

Reference	Population	Design	Intervention	Outcome Measures
May et al. (18)	45 NUD patients	Randomized, parallel, double-blind	Enteroplant (90 mg peppermint oil + 50 mg caraway oil tid) vs. placebo for 4 weeks	Patient scoring of pain intensity and frequency on Clinical Global Impression Scale
Carling et al. (20)	40 IBS patients	Randomized, cross-over	Colpermin (0.2–0.4 mL tid peppermint oil) vs. placebo for 2 weeks	Symptom score Global improvement in symptoms
Dew et al. (21)	29 IBS patients	Randomized, double-blind, cross-over	Elanco (0.2–0.4 mL peppermint oil tid) vs. placebo for 2 weeks	Symptom score Global improvement in symptoms
Lech et al. (22)	47 IBS patients	Randomized, parallel, double-blind	0.2 mL peppermint oil in enteric capsules TID vs. placebo for 4 weeks	Symptom score Global improvement in symptoms
Nash et al. (23)	41 IBS patients	Randomized, double-blind, cross-over	Colpermin (0.4 mL peppermint oil tid) vs. placebo for 2 weeks	Symptom score Global improvement in symptoms
Rees et al. (24)	18 IBS patients	Randomized, double-blind, cross-over	Elanco (0.2–0.4 mL peppermint oil) TID vs. placebo for 3 weeks	Symptom score Global improvement in symptoms
Tatsuta et al. (25)	42 NUD patients	Randomized, parallel (blinding unclear)	TJ-43* tid vs. placebo for 1 week	Gastric emptying measured by acetaminophen absorption Symptom score
Thamlikitkul et al. (33)	116 NUD patients	Randomized, parallel (blinding unclear)	*Curcura domestica* (dried rhizome) 500 mg bid vs. placebo vs. cascara 130 mg bid for 1 week	Global improvement in symptoms Patient satisfaction with medication
Bensoussan et al. (28)	116 IBS patients	Randomized, parallel, double-blind	Standard Chinese Herbal 3 tablets† 5×/d vs. Individualized Chinese Herbal 3 tablets 5×/d vs. placebo for 16 weeks	Bowel symptom scores Global improvement in symptoms
Yadav et al. (34)	214 IBS patients	Randomized, parallel, double-blind	Ayurvedic preparation vs. clinidium bromide (2.5 mg) + chlordiazopoxide (5 mg) vs. placebo for 2 weeks	Symptom severity score Global response to therapy

IBS = irritable bowel syndrome; NUD = nonulcer dyspepsia.

* TJ-43 contains 0.74 g *Atractylodis lancue rhizoma*, 0.74 g Ginseng, 0.74 g *Pinelliae* hair, 0.74 g Hoden, 0.37 g *Zizyohi fructus*, 0.37 g *Aurantii nobilis perocarpium*, 0.20 g *Glycirrhizae* radix, and 0.10 gm *Zingiberis rhizona*.

† Standard Chinese Herbal Medicine tablet contains *Codonopsis pilosulae*, radix (7%); *Agastaches seu pogostemi*, herba (4.5%); *Ledebourieilae sesloidis*, radix (3%); *Coicis lachryma-jobi*, semen (7%); *Bupleurum chinense* (4.5%); *Artemesiae capillaris*, herba (13%); *Atractylodis macrocephalae*, rhizoma (4.5%); *Fraxini*, cortex (4.5%); *Poriae cocos, Sclerotium hoelen* (4.5%); *Angelicae dahuricae*, radix (2%); *Plantaginis*, semen (4.5%); *Phellodenari*, cortex (4.5%); *Glycyrrhizae uralensis*, radix (4.5%); *Paeoniae lactiflorae*, radix (3%); *Saussureae seu vladiminrae*, radix (3%); *Coptidis*, rhizoma (3%); *Schisandrae*, fructus (7%).

Table 10.4   Psychotherapy in Nonulcer Dyspepsia and Irritable Bowel Syndrome

Reference	Population	Design	Intervention	Outcome Measures
Haug et al. (41)	100 NUD patients	Randomized	10 50-minute sessions of cognitive psychotherapy vs. no treatment	Assessment of NUD symptoms and generic quality of life before and after treatment
Mine et al. (42)	194 consecutive NUD patients	Randomized	Combination of 8 weeks of medical, psychiatric, and psychotherapeutic treatment vs. medical therapy alone	Assessment of NUD symptoms and generic quality of life; effect on ADL before and after treatment
Bennett et al. (43)	24 IBS patients	Randomized	Eight 1-hour sessions of individual behavioral therapy vs. medical therapy	Self- and family-member assessment before and after treatment
Blanchard et al. (study 1) (44)	30 IBS patients	Randomized	12 1-hour sessions of multicomponent therapy vs. attention-placebo vs. symptom monitoring	Symptom diaries and visual analog scales before and after treatment
Blanchard et al. (study 2) (45)	115 IBS patients	Randomized	12 1-hour seessions of multicomponent therapy vs. attention-placebo vs. symptom monitoring	Symptom diaries and visual analog scales before and after treatment
Corney et al. (46)	42 IBS patients	Randomized	Six to 15 1-hour sessions of behavioral therapy vs. medical therapy	Self-reporting of IBS symptoms
Greene et al. (47)	20 IBS patients	Randomized	10 1-hour sessions of individual cognitive therapy vs. symptom monitoring	Symptom diaries visual analog scales before and after treatment
Guthrie et al. (48)	102 consecutive IBS patients	Randomized	12 45-minute sessions of dynamic psychotherapy vs. six 30-minute sessions of supportive listening plus medical therapy	Physician and patient severity assessment based on Likert scale and patient maintained IBS symptom diary
Harvey et al. (49)	33 IBS patients	Randomized	Four 40-minute sessions of individual hypnotherapy vs. group hypnotherapy	Daily IBS symptom diary
Lynch et al. (50)	21 IBS patients	Randomized	Eight 2-hour sessions of behavioral therapy vs. symptom monitoring	Daily IBS symptom diary
Rumsey (51)	37 consecutive IBS patients	Randomized	Six 1.5-hour sessions of group stress management vs. psychiatric medical therapy	Semi-structured interview and self-assessment
Shaw et al. (52)	35 IBS patients	Randomized	Six 40-minute sessions of stress management program vs. antispasmodic therapy	Self-assessment before and after treatment
Whorwell et al. (53)	30 IBS patients	Randomized	Seven 30-minute sessions of hypnotherapy over 3 months vs. supportive discussion and placebo	Independent investigator assessment and visual analog scales of IBS symptoms and quality of life
Blanchard et al. (54)	16 IBS patients	Randomized	10 sessions of progressive muscle relaxation vs. symptom monitoring	IBS symptom diaries before and after treatment
Svedlund et al. (55)	101 IBS patients	Randomized	10 1-hour sessions of dynamic psychotherapy vs. medical therapy	Semi-structured interviews and self-rating of symptoms

ADL = activities of daily living; IBS = irritable bowel syndrome; NUD = nonulcer dyspepsia.

Results

Herbal Medicine and Traditional Chinese Herbal Medicine

Several formulations of peppermint oil have been studied for the treatment of NUD and IBS. Peppermint oil, which is obtained by the steam distillation of flowering *Menta X piperita L*, has been reported to have antispasmodic effects on the gastrointestinal tract (*see* Table 10.2). Only one randomized controlled trial (RCT) (18) has examined the efficacy of peppermint oil in the treatment of NUD (*see* Table 10.3). In this trial, more patients using Enteroplant (peppermint oil 90 mg and caraway oil 50 mg) had improvement of their pain symptoms compared with patients using placebo (89.5% vs. 45%, respectively; p = 0.015), and more patients using Enteroplant had improvement in a Clinical Global Impression scale compared with patients using placebo (94.5% vs. 55%, respectively; p = 0.008). No significant difference in adverse events was recorded for Enteroplant compared with placebo.

Peppermint oil also has been studied among IBS patients in one meta-analysis (19) and five RCTs (20–24). All five RCTs were double-blind placebo-controlled trials (*see* Table 10.3) and formed the meta-analysis. With global improvement of symptoms as the end point, the meta-analysis demonstrated that IBS patients using peppermint oil were eight times more likely to demonstrate improvement compared with placebo patients. No significant differences in adverse events were recorded for peppermint oil compared with placebo in any of the RCTs. However, heartburn, nausea, vomiting, blurred vision, and flatulence were all reported in patients using peppermint oil.

Several formulations of traditional Chinese herbs also have been studied in patients with NUD and IBS. Only one RCT (25) has examined the efficacy of traditional Chinese herbs for the treatment of NUD. In this trial (*see* Table 10.3), patients using a specific combination of eight herbs (TJ-43) had improved gastric emptying significantly by using a serum acetaminophen absorption technique. Patients using Chinese herbs also demonstrated significant improvement in epigastric fullness, heartburn, belching, and nausea compared with patients receiving placebo. No significant differences in side effects were identified between study groups. These findings also have been supported by several nonrandomized trials (26,27). The use of traditional Chinese herbs also has been studied among IBS patients. In one well-designed trial by Bensoussan and coworkers (28), IBS patients were randomized to receive an individualized combination of Chinese herbs, a traditional combination of Chinese herbs, or placebo. More patients given either individualized or traditional Chinese herbs demonstrated improvement than did placebo patients for bowel symptoms scores (42%, 44%, and 19% improvement, respectively; p = 0.03) and for global improvement in symptoms (64%, 76%, 33% improvement, respectively; p = 0.007). Adverse effects were not significantly different between treatment groups. Several additional randomized trials (29–32), all described in Chinese language medical journals, reportedly support these results; however, these non-English articles were not reviewed for this publication.

Two additional randomized trials (33,34) of herbal medicine also were retrieved. In one trial (34), NUD patients in Thailand were given a preparation of dried rhizome (*Curcura domestica*), which is frequently used in Chinese herbal medicine (*see* Table 10.3). More patients receiving this preparation experienced significant improvement in symptoms than did patients receiving placebo (87% and 53%, respectively; p = 0.008). In the second trial (34), IBS patients in India received Ayurvedic preparation of *Aegle marmelos* Correa plus *Bacopa monniere* (*see* Table 10.3). More patients receiving this preparation demonstrated symptom improvement than did patients receiving placebo (65% and 33%, respectively; $p < 0.05$).

Two caveats about methodology should be considered when assessing the results of herbal medicine trials. First, none of these trials used validated questionnaires to assess the improvement of symptoms. Second, except for one 16-week trial (28), all of the trials were 2 to 6 weeks in duration, and the improvements associated with these alternative treatments may wane with prolonged use (especially if part of the treatment benefit resulted from a placebo effect). Nevertheless, given the current data about efficacy and side effects, peppermint oil and traditional Chinese herbal medicine may be reasonable treatment options for NUD patients who have not responded to more conventional treatments.

Acupuncture and Acupressure

Previous reviews indicate that acupuncture does affect gastrointestinal motility, electrical activity, gastric secretion, and cytoprotection in animals and humans (35). The proposed mechanism of action, similar to the well-documented pain-modification qualities of acupuncture, is via somatic afferent stimulation at various levels of the central nervous system, inducing a variable autonomic nervous system response primarily through neural opioid peptide pathways (35). Several controlled animal studies show that the administration of nalaxone inhibits acupuncture-mediated changes in motility and gastric acid secretion (36,37), whereas administration of morphine mimics such changes (38). However, it remains unproven that the effect of acupuncture on the gastrointestinal system is anything more than a response to a nonspecific stress.

To our knowledge, there have been no randomized or observational trials examining the use of acupuncture or acupressure as a treatment modality for NUD. Zhenzhi and Deyou (39) did examine the use of moxibustion (acupuncture with the addition of warmth over the acupoints) in a "pseudorandomized" study of 137 patients with acute "gastric spasm" and "intestinal spasm." Ninety-seven patients were treated with one session of moxibustion and 40 control patients received 0.5-mg intramuscular atropine injections. In this trial, patients treated with moxibustion had a higher rate of symptomatic relief (93.8% and 77.5%, respectively; p not available) and a lower rate of pain relapse within 24 hours (6.6% and 23%, respectively; p not available).

Chan and coworkers (40) examined the use of acupuncture as a therapy for IBS in 1997. They used a four-point Likert scale for patient grading of gastrointestinal symptoms, including pain, bloating, and stool frequency. They also used a 10-point visual analog scale to assess patients' own sense of well-being. In their small ($n = 7$), nonrandomized trial, they found that acupuncture resulted in statistically significant pre- and post-treatment improvements in the patients' sense of well-being (6.6 [±1.2] and 2.6 [±1.1], respectively; $p < 0.002$) and bloating (1.6 [±0.7] vs. 1.1 [±0.9], respectively; p < 0.001). There were no significant pre- and post-treatment changes in bowel frequency (1.4 [±1.1] and 1.3 [±0.9], respectively; $p > 0.05$) or discomfort (1.5 [±0.8] and 1.3 [±1.0], respectively; $p > 0.05$).

Before any definitive conclusion can be reached about the use of acupuncture for dyspepsia, more systematic, carefully designed, rigorously controlled human studies are needed. Thus far, most of the evidence that supports acupuncture as an accepted therapeutic modality is anecdotal at best, and no recommendation for or against its use in the treatment of functional bowel disorders can be made.

Psychotherapy and Hypnotherapy

There have been two RCTs (41,42) evaluating the use of psychotherapy for NUD (*see* Table 10.4). Both reported significant benefits compared with placebo or standard medical therapy in NUD symptoms. In one trial (41), patients underwent ten sessions of cognitive-based psychotherapy compared with no treatment to determine if there was any difference in dyspeptic symptoms. The investigators noted a statistically significant greater reduction in epigastric pain, nausea, bloating, diarrhea, and constipation (numerical results not available; $p < 0.05$ for all analyses). In the second trial (42), patients who received a combination of psychiatric, psychological, and medical therapies experienced statistically significant improvement in their NUD symptoms compared with patients that received medical therapy alone (numerical results not available; $p < 0.0001$). Patients were classified as having "serious NUD" if their symptoms preempted work or study. A significantly larger proportion of patients diagnosed with "serious NUD" treated with the combined therapy were able to return to work or study compared with the controls (74% and 5%, respectively; $p < 0.0001$). Notably, patients with "serious NUD" were more likely to be classified as having a psychiatric illness compared with subjects with "mild NUD" (numerical results not available; $p < 0.0001$).

In contrast to the paucity of psychotherapeutic trials for NUD, one of the most popular emerging treatments for IBS has been the development of psychotherapeutic approaches to the condition. Thirteen randomized studies have examined the role of various types of psychotherapy in the treatment of IBS (43–55) (*see* Table 10.4). Seven of these studies reported statistically significant improvement in IBS symptoms of those patients treated with a psychotherapeutic approach compared with placebo or traditional medical therapy alone (47,48,50,52–55). Five studies did not report a significant improvement (43–46,49), but three of these did report a trend toward improvement in IBS symptomatology compared with baseline measures after a psychotherapeutic approach was used (44–46). One trial did not report whether or not psychotherapy was superior to control therapy (51). Overall, patients with less severe IBS symptoms and lesser degrees of psychological disturbance tend to respond more favorably to this type of treatment. Younger age and a shorter duration of symptoms also seem to be associated with a better response to psychotherapeutic approaches. Cognitive-based behavioral psychotherapy is the most widely studied approach.

Hypnotherapy has not been evaluated as a treatment modality for NUD, but there has been one RCT examining the use of hypnotherapy for IBS (53). This trial randomized 30 severe, refractory IBS patients to treatment with hypnotherapy compared with a control group treated with supportive psychotherapy. Supportive psychotherapy consisted of a discussion of symptoms and an exploration of possible contributory emotional problems or stressors. Symptoms were detailed by the patients on diary cards with numerical gradations of symptom severity. At the end of the 3-month trial, the patients in the hypnotherapy group had significantly greater improvements in their scores for IBS and general well-being compared with those in the control group (numerical results not available; $p < 0.0001$). These findings, as well as improvements in absenteeism and primary care use, were supported by a later nonrandomized case-control trial that demonstrated a beneficial role of hypnosis as a therapy for IBS compared with both placebo and traditional medical treatment (56).

Although multiple controlled studies have reported significant benefits of psychotherapy or psychotherapeutic approaches to IBS compared with placebo or standard medical therapy, many of these studies suffer from significant methodologic flaws (Table 10.5). In 1996, Talley and coworkers (57) reviewed the published trials of psychological therapy for IBS to date. They found significant methodologic limitations in nearly every study reviewed. Common limitations included the lack of consecutive subjects (43–47,49,50, 52–55), an inadequate or unclear definition of IBS (43–45,51,54), poor description of baseline characteristics (43–45,49,51), and generally small sample sizes that limited the statistical power of these studies. Nevertheless, if one accepts that the overlap between IBS and NUD is 35% to 40%, as suggested, cognitive-behavioral therapy may benefit patients with functional bowel disorders, especially those refractory to conventional treatment.

Conclusions

The management of NUD may frustrate the most skilled clinicians. Given the limited benefit of traditional pharmaceuticals and the chronic discomfort associated with this disorder, it is not surprising that many NUD patients turn to alternative therapies. However, the efficacy of these alternative therapies should be demonstrated in well-designed randomized trials before these treatments are broadly recommended. Unfortunately, trials of these therapies have been marked by inadequate randomization, lack of blinding, brief study duration, and the use of nonvalidated questionnaires (28). In the future, the methodologies of alternative medicine trials should meet previously described criteria for well-designed trials (57) (*see* Table 10.5).

Although the available data about alternative therapies are limited, these data indicate that peppermint oil, Chinese herbal medicine, and cognitive psychotherapy are beneficial for functional bowel disorders. These interventions do not seem to have significant adverse effects compared

---

Table 10.5   Recommendations for Trials Testing Psychologic Treatment for Irritable Bowel Syndrome

---

- Describe the study population; consider enrolling a medical treatment-resistant population.

- Use a consensus-based operational definition of IBS.

- Enroll a consecutive sample.

- Enroll a sample size large enough for adequate power.

- Record information on those who refuse to enter the study.

- Randomize patients and describe the method used to randomize.

- Compare pretreatment characteristics of the groups, including IBS symptoms and psychological factors.

- Include groups to control for expectancy, nonspecific factors, and standard medical treatment.

- Ensure blinding of outcome assessors.

- Ensure IBS outcome measures are reliable, valid, and sensitive to change.

- Assess and account for concurrent drug use.

- Measure relevant symptoms and psychological changes pre- to posttreatment.

- Assess compliance with treatment.

- Measure dropout numbers and characteristics.

- Conduct an intention-to-treat analysis.

- Conduct long-term follow-up of all groups.

- Define clinical significance a priori.

IBS = irritable bowel syndrome.
Adapted from Talley, NJ, Owen BK, Boyce P, et al. Psychological treatments for irritable bowel syndrome: a critique of controlled treatment trials. *Am J Gastroenterol.* 1996;91:277–86.

with placebo. Therefore, the use of these therapies seems to be a reasonable alternative for NUD patients that have already failed conventional treatments.

■   ■   ■

Key Points

- Because conventional medical treatments for NUD often fail to relieve symptoms, patients with this disorder often turn to alternative medicine therapies.

- Because herbal medicine is not regulated by the Food and Drug Administration, adverse reactions resulting from contaminated or improperly processed herbal products have been reported. To help avoid adverse reactions, one should review the product labeling carefully and purchase only those herbal medicines produced by reputable U.S. manufacturers.

- Peppermint oil and traditional Chinese herbal medicine may be considered for patients with NUD who are refractory to conventional treatment, although improvement in symptoms may wane with prolonged use.

- The results of acupuncture efficacy studies are inconclusive; therefore, this treatment cannot be recommended.

- Cognitive-behavioral therapy may be beneficial in patients with NUD.

■   ■   ■

REFERENCES

1. **Panel on Definition and Description at the CAM Research Methodology Conference.** Defining and describing complementary and alternative medicine. *Alt Ther.* 1997;3:49–57.

2. **Eisenberg DM, Davis RB, Ettner SL, et al.** Trends in alternative medicine use in the United States, 1990–97. *JAMA.* 1998;280:1569–75.

3. **Davidoff F.** Weighing the alternatives: lessons from the paradoxes of alternative medicine. *Ann Intern Med.* 1998;129:1068–70.

4. **Astin JA.** Why patients use alternative medicine: results of a national study. *JAMA.* 1998;279:1548–53.

5. **Smart HL, Mayberry JF, Atkinson M.** Alternative medicine consultations and remedies in patients with irritable bowel syndrome. *Gut.* 1986;27:826–8.

6. **Talley NJ and the Working Team for Functional Gastroduodenal Disorders.** Functional gastroduodenal disorders. In Drossman DA (ed). *The Functional Gastrointestinal Disorders.* Boston: Little, Brown; 1994:71–113.

7. **Muller J, Clauson K.** Pharmaceutical considerations of common herbal medicine. *Am J Manag Care.* 1997;3:1753–70.

8. **Millman C.** Natural disasters. *Men's Health.* 1999;6:90–5.

9. **Chan TYK, Critchley JAJH.** Usage and adverse effects of Chinese herbal medicine. *Hum Exp Tox.* 1996;15:5–12.

10. **Rosenthal M.** Philosophy of Chinese Herbal Medicine. Center for Complementary and Alternative Medicine of Columbia. www.camcentercolumbia, 1998.

11. **Foley WT.** Chinese medicine: the ancient art. *J Pract Nurs.* 1977;27:14,15,33.

12. **Helms JM.** An overview of medical acupuncture. *Alt Ther.* 1998;4:35–45.

13. **Vincent CA, Richardson PH.** Acupuncture for some common disorders: a review of evaluative research. *J R Coll Gen Practit.* 1987;37:77–81.

14. **Spring M.** The practical aspects of acupuncture. *Bull NY Acad Med.* 1975:914–21.

15. **Talley NK, Owen BK, Boyce P, Patterson K.** Psychological treatments for irritable bowel syndrome: a critique of controlled clinical trials. *Am J Gastroenterol.* 1996;91:277–86.

16. **Talley NL, Fung LH, Gilligan IG, et al.** Association of anxiety, neuroticism, and depression with dyspepsia of unknown cause. *Gastroenterology.* 1986;90:886–92.

17. **Talley NJ, Piper DW.** The association between nonulcer dyspepsia and other gastrointestinal disorders. *Scand J Gastroenterol.* 1985;20:896–900.

18. **May B, Kuntz HD, Kieser M, Kohler S.** Efficacy of a fixed peppermint oil/caraway oil combination in non-ulcer dyspepsia. *Arzneimittelforschung.* 1996;46:1149–53.

19. **Pittler, MH, Ernst E.** Peppermint oil for irritable bowel syndrome: a critical review and meta-analysis. *Am J Gastroenterol.* 1998;93:1131–5.

20. **Carling I, Svedberg LE, Hulten S.** Short-term treatment of the irritable bowel syndrome: a placebo-controlled trial of peppermint oil against hyoscyamine. *OPMEAR.* 1989;34:55–57.

21. **Dew MJ, Evans BK, Rhodes J.** Peppermint oil for the irritable bowel syndrome: a multicentre trial. *Br J Clin Pract.* 1984;38:394–8.

22. **Lech Y, Olesen KM, Hey H, et al.** Treatment of irritable bowel syndrome with peppermint oil: a double-blind study with a placebo. *Ugeskr Laeger.* 1988;150:2388–9.

23. **Nash P, Gould SR, Barnardo DE.** Peppermint oil does not relieve the pain of irritable bowel syndrome. *Br J Clin Pract.* 1986;40:292–3.

24. **Rees WDW, Evans BK, Rhodes J.** Treating the irritable bowel syndrome with peppermint oil. *BMJ.* 1979;2:835–6.

25. **Tatsuta M, Iishi H.** Effect of treatment with Liu-Jun-Zi-Tang (TJ-43) on gastric emptying and gastrointestinal symptoms in dyspeptic patients. *Aliment Pharmacol Ther.* 1993;7:459–62.

26. **Harasaw S, Miwa T.** Chronic effects of Tsumura Rikkunshi-to (TJ-43) on gastric emptying in nonulcer dyspepsia and a study of its clinical effects. *Shyokaki-ka.* 1990;12:215–22.

27. **Kawamura S, Ariyama S, Tanabe M, et al.** Clinical effect of Tsumura Rikkunshi-to (TJ-43) on the upper abdominal symptoms. *Kampo-Igaku.* 1990;14:14–20.

28. **Bensoussan A, Talley N, Hing M, Menzies R, Guo A, Ngu M.** Treatment of irritable bowel syndrome with Chinese herbal medicine: a randomized controlled trial. *JAMA.* 1998;280:1585–9.

29. **Xu RL.** Clinical realizations during the diagnosis and treatment of 55 cases of irritable bowel syndrome. *Shanxi J Tradit Chin Med.* 1995;11:10–1.

30. **Chen DZ.** Tong Xie Yao Fang with additions in treating 106 cases of irritable bowel syndrome. *Nanjing Med Univ J.* 1995;15:924.

31. **Shi ZQ.** Combination treatment of Chinese and Western medicine for 30 cases of irritable bowel syndrome. *Chin J Integrated Tradit West Med.* 1989;9:241.

32. **Liu ZK.** Chinese herbal medicine treatment for 120 cases of irritable bowel syndrome. *Chin J Integrated Tradit West Med.* 1990;10:615.

33. **Thamlikitkul V, Dechatiwongse T, Chantrakul C, et al.** Randomized double-blind study of *Curcuma domestica* for dyspepsia. *J Med Assoc Thai.* 1989;72: 614–20.

34. **Yadav SK, Jain AK, Tripathi SN, Gupta JP.** Irritable bowel syndrome: therapeutic evaluation of indigenous drugs. *Indian J Med Res.* 1989;90:496–503.

35. **Li Y, Tougas G, Chiverton SG, Hunt RH.** The effect of acupuncture on gastrointestinal function and disorders. *Am J Gastroenterol.* 1992;87:1372–81.

36. **Jiang SL, Liu ZM, Sun GR.** Acupuncture at Zusanli and gastrointestinal motility: the specificity of Zusanli and its afferent pathways. *Abstracts of the International Symposium of Acupuncture.* Beijing; Nov 1987:127.

37. **Sodipo JOA, Falaiye JM.** Acupuncture and gastric acid studies. *Am J Chin Med.* 1979;7:356–61.

38. **Lin YL, Chen SM, Li ZH.** Effects of microinjection of nalaxone into the dorsal part of the cat medulla oblongata on the antral contraction induced by acupuncture. *Acta Physiol Sinica.* 1984;36:49–55.

39. **Zhenzhi S, Deyou Z.** 97 cases of gastrointestinal spasm treated with moxibustion. *J Tradit Chin Med.* 1991;11:110–1.

40. **Chan J, Carr I, Mayberry JF.** The role of acupuncture in the treatment of irritable bowel syndrome: a pilot study. *Hepatogastroenterology.* 1997;44:1328–30.

41. **Haug TT, Wilhelmsen I, Svebak S, et al.** Psychotherapy in functional dyspepsia. *J Psyhosom Res.* 1994;38:735–44.

42. **Mine K, Kanazawa F, Hosoi M, et al.** Treating nonulcer dyspepsia considering both functional disorders of the digestive system and psychiatric conditions. *Dig Dis Sci.* 1998;43:1241–7.

43. **Bennett P, Wilkinson SA.** Comparison of pyschological and medical treatment of the irritable bowel syndrome. *Br J Clin Psychol.* 1985;24:215–6.

44. **Blanchard EB, Schwarz SP, Suls JM, et al.** Two controlled evaluations of multicomponent psychological treatment of irritable bowel syndrome (study 1). *Behav Res Ther.* 1992;30:175–89.

45. **Blanchard EB, Schwarz SP, Suls JM, et al.** Two controlled evaluations of multicomponent psychological treatment of irritable bowel syndrome (study 2). *Behav Res Ther.* 1992;30:175–89.

46. **Corney RH, Stanton R, Newell R et al.** Behavioural psychotherapy in the treatment of irritable bowel syndrome. *J Psychosom Res.* 1991;35:461–9.

47. **Greene B, Blanchard EB.** Cognitive therapy for irritable bowel syndrome. *J Consult Clin Psychol.* 1994;62:576–82.

48. **Guthrie E, Creed F, Dawson D et al.** A randomized controlled trial of psychotherapy in patients with refractory irritable bowel syndrome. *Br J Psychiatry.* 1993;163:315–21.

49. **Harvey RF, Hinton RA, Gunary RM, et al.** Individual and group hypnotherapy in treatment of refractory irritable bowel syndrome. *Lancet.* 1989;1:424–5.

50. **Lynch PM, Zamble EA.** Controlled behavioral treatment study of irritable bowel syndrome. *Behav Ther.* 1987;20:509–23.

51. **Rumsey N.** Group stress management programmes vs. pharmacological treatment in the treatment of irritable bowel syndrome. In Heaton KW, Creed F, Goeting NLM (eds). *Towards Confident Management of Irritable Bowel Syndrome: Current Approaches.* London: Duphar Medical Relations; 1991:33–9.

52. **Shaw G, Sriviatava ED, Sadlier M, et al.** Stress management for irritable bowel syndrome: a controlled trial. *Digestion.* 1991;50:36–42.

53. **Whorwell PJ, Prior A, Farragher EB.** Controlled trial of hypnotherapy in the treatment of severe refractory irritable bowel syndrome. *Lancet.* 1984;2:1232–4.

54. **Blanchard EB, Greene B, Scharff L, et al.** Relaxation training as a treatment for irritable bowel syndrome. *Biofeedback Self Regul.* 1993;18:125–32.

55. **Svedlund J, Sjödin I, Ottosson JO, et al.** Controlled study of psychotherapy in irritable bowel syndrome. *Lancet.* 1983;2:589–91.

56. **Houghton LA, Heyman DJ, Whorwell PJ.** Symptomatology, quality of life, and economic features of irritable bowel syndrome: the effect of hypnotherapy. *Aliment Pharmacol Ther.* 1996;10:91–5.

57. **Talley, NJ, Owen BK, Boyce P, et al.** Psychological treatments for irritable bowel syndrome: a critique of controlled treatment trials. *Am J Gastroenterol.* 1996;91: 277–86.

Clinical Vignettes

Patient with History of Treated *Helicobacter pylori* Infection and Recurrent Dyspepsia

A man 41 years of age with a previous, well-documented peptic ulcer presents with complaints of heartburn and indigestion. He had treatment for *Helicobacter pylori* 1 year ago and has not knowingly had a recurrence of his previously symptomatic ulcer. Over the past year, the patient has gained 10 pounds, has been eating well, and has had no abdominal complaints whatsoever. Over the past several months, however, he has noted increasing heartburn, in particular after eating. The location of the discomfort is in the substernal area and is frequently aggravated postprandially and occasionally with recumbency. He also has regurgitation. The patient denies symptoms of dysphagia, odynophagia, and has not had clinical signs of overt bleeding, weight loss, or other systemic complaints.

■ QUESTION

What is the patient's most likely cause of heartburn? Should he be retested for *H. pylori*?

■ COMMENTS

This patient presents with a fairly classic description of gastroesophageal reflux after treatment for *H. pylori* infection. There is growing evidence that in a significant portion of patients infected with *H. pylori*, GERD symptoms develop following *H. pylori* eradication (1,2). There are a number of possible mechanisms that might account for rebound reflux after *H. pylori* cure. Ammonia produced by *H. pylori* , including infection at the gastric cardia or in a hiatal hernia, could potentially help neutralize acid that refluxes into the esophagus. This buffering effect is lost after *H. pylori* cure. Because corpus gastritis is associated with diminished acid secretion, healing of corpus gastritis after *H. pylori* cure also may result in an increase in acid secretory capability. Additionally, it is speculated that *H. pylori* infection may increase alkaline duodenogastric reflux. Some evidence suggests that *H. pylori* also changes nitric oxide synthase and may have the capacity to inhibit the acid secretion via a nitric oxide–mediated pathway. Labenz and coworkers (1) suggest that weight gain is an independent risk factor for posteradication reflux, but the role of obesity per se in promoting GERD is still somewhat controversial.

H. pylori status seems to influence the efficacy of antisecretory therapy, in particular proton-pump inhibitors (PPIs). There are several possible reasons for this. One reason is that *H. pylori* infection causes a lessened acid-secretion state. Also, *H. pylori* infection affects gastrin levels, stimulating parietal cells—a process necessary for PPIs to inactivate the H^+-K^+ ATPase pump (3).

In the patient who has received adequate treatment for *H. pylori*, the chance of relapse is less than 5% to 10%. Treatment with a PPI-based triple therapy (with combination antibiotics) should diminish the chance for potential relapse considerably. However, many patients may have been treated before standard regimens for *H. pylori* were established. Similarly, recommendations for extended treatment up to 2 weeks have been accepted as standard only in the past few years. Accordingly, patients who had not received adequate treatment clearly may be at risk for *H. pylori* relapse.

■ CONCLUSION

In this patient, typical symptoms of reflux are evident. The patient has postprandial discomfort, regurgitation, and substernal burning, all of which represent a fairly classic history of GERD symptoms. Accordingly, directed treatment for GERD in the absence of diagnostic testing is the most appropriate strategy.

REFERENCES

1. **Labenz J, Blum AL, Payerdorffer E, et al.** Curing *Helicobacter pylori* infection in patients with duodenal ulcer may provoke reflux oesophagitis. *Gastroenterology.* 1997;112:1442–7.

2. **O'Connor HJ.** *Helicobacter pylori* and gastro-oesophageal reflux disease: clinical implications and management (Review). *Aliment Pharmacol Ther.* 1999;13:117–27.

3. **Labenz J.** Does *Helicobacter pylori* affect the management of gastroesophageal reflux disease? *Am J Gastroenterol.* 1999;94:867–9.

Young Woman with Bloating Dyspepsia

A woman 26 years of age presents for evaluation of abdominal discomfort and bloating. She has had a several-year history of abdominal symptoms with prominent gaseous distention, intermittent belching, rectal flatus, and occasional epigastric pain. She has mild early satiety and sustained weight loss but no postprandial nausea or vomiting. She denies systemic complaints, fevers, chills, sweats, and arthralgias. There is no history of thyroid or diabetic disease, rheumatologic syndrome, or neuromuscular disease. She is on no regular medications. The physical examination is normal, revealing a well-seeming young woman. Focus on the abdominal examination shows no evidence of organomegaly or abdominal distention. There is no succussion splash. Laboratory profile includes a complete blood count with differential, which is normal. No other laboratory tests have been performed.

■ QUESTION

What is the differential diagnosis and the most appropriate therapy?

■ COMMENTS

This patient presents a fairly typical history for a dysmotility syndrome associated with dyspepsia. It is estimated that up to half of nonulcer dyspepsia patients have some form of gastric emptying delay or abnormal postprandial antral motility (1). The relationship between gastric emptying abnormalities and reported symptoms is somewhat unclear. The differential diagnosis in this patient should focus on dysmotility, given the symptoms of early satiety. Less likely, this represents an outlet obstructive symptom because she did not have severe postprandial nausea or vomiting. The abdominal bloating certainly is compatible with dysmotility or a functionally related disorder. Some patients also may have aerophagia, a self-propagating cycle of abdominal bloating followed by air swallowing to induce belching that, in turn, is followed by worsened bloating.

The best diagnostic and management strategy for patients with a suspected motility disorder should be directed somewhat by the associated symptoms (2). For example, this patient does not have symptoms of weight loss, nausea, vomiting, or other alarm symptoms, so it would be reasonable to try empirical therapy with prokinetic agents such as cisapride before em-barking on more directed testing. In older patients or patients with new on-set of symptoms, a more directed and aggressive diagnostic strategy (e.g., early endoscopy) needs to be performed. As always, any diagnostic testing should be coupled with good clinical judgment. Persistence despite empir-ical therapy with a prokinetic agent warrants further diagnostic testing, such as gastric-emptying study and motility assessment. Endoscopy with possible gastric emptying evaluation should be considered when these methods fail.

The patient has been placed on cisapride 10 mg at one half-hour before every meal and at bedtime. Her abdominal bloating discomfort continues to improve; in particular, she experiences less early satiety and postprandial complaint. At 3-month follow-up, the patient has improved dramatically.

CONCLUSION

In patients with symptoms suggestive of gastric dys-motility (e.g., early satiety, potential fullness), the dif-ferential diagnosis should focus appropriately on a motility disorder. Empirical therapy with a prokinetic agent is the treatment of choice.

REFERENCES

1. **Stanghellini V, Tosetti C, Paternico A, et al.** Risky indicators that delayed gastric emptying of solids in patients with functional dyspepsia. *Gastroenterology.* 1996;110:1036–42.
2. **Fisher RS, Parkman HP.** Management of nonulcer dyspepsia. *N Engl J Med.* 1998;339:1376–81.

Middle-Aged Man
with Long-Standing Heartburn

A man 49 years of age presents with long-standing acid indigestion. He has a 10-to 15-year history of intermittent regurgitant symptoms. Over the past several months, he has had increased frequency of symptoms that now occur on a daily basis. His symptoms are aggravated postprandially and also are associated with recumbency, in particular if he lies on his right side. He has not had associated weight loss, and he denies dysphagia or odynophagia. He is on no medications other than as-needed antacids and over-the-counter H_2-receptor antagonists (H2RAs), which have provided only marginal benefit. On physical examination, he seems to be a healthy 49-year-old white man. Oropharyngeal examination is notable for somewhat poor dentition, but his physical examination is otherwise unremarkable.

■ QUESTION

What are the most appropriate diagnostic and therapeutic approaches to this patient?

This patient presented with a fairly typical history for gastroesophageal reflux disease (GERD). The diagnostic approach in this patient was to treat GERD without directed testing in the absence of alarm symptoms (e.g., nausea, vomiting, weight loss, bleeding, obstructive symptoms of dysphagia). In this case, given his daily symptoms and previous use of H2RAs, the most appropriate treatment is to begin with a proton-pump inhibitor (PPI) and reserve early diagnostic testing for a failure to respond or for the presence of alarm symptoms. In the absence of a typical history for GERD, the initial diagnostic approach might favor earlier endoscopy. In this case, the diagnostic endoscopy was done not to establish the diagnosis of GERD but rather to evaluate for possible Barrett's esophagus, given the patient's chronic reflux symptoms.

Patients with chronic reflux symptoms for more than 5 years should be considered for Barrett's esophagus screening. The highest profile for Barrett's-related cancers is white men in their fifth decade of life. Accordingly, this population clearly warrants diagnostic testing with one-time endoscopy for possible Barrett's esophagus and a surveillance regimen if Barrett's is identified. It is the preferred approach to treat patients with PPIs before investigating for possible Barrett's esophagus. Active erosive or ulcerative esophagitis can mask areas of columnar epithelium and potentially lead to sampling error. Accordingly, it is better to heal any mucosal inflammatory response to allow more directed biopsies in areas of suspected Barrett's epithelium. In the present patient, this led to establishing a diagnosis after the patient came back on therapy and received an elective endoscopy.

There are two interesting side notes. First, this patient experienced a worsening of his reflux symptoms when he was recumbent on his right side, a position that has been shown to be worse than lying on the left side in patients with chronic reflux. In addition, the patient did have severe dental deterioration that may have been a manifestation of gastroesophageal reflux with etching of the dental enamel. Dental deterioration in adults should always raise GERD as a differential concern.

The patient was placed on a PPI for presumed GERD. At 8-week follow-up, the patient is without symptoms. Upper endoscopy is performed at that time and shows evidence of Barrett's esophagus and intestinal metaplasia. Accordingly, the patient has been entered into a surveillance regimen for follow-up endoscopies.

CONCLUSION

Recently, tremendous attention has been given to the symptom of heartburn, which has been gaining some respect. The extremely well-planned and -executed epidemiologic study performed by Lagergren and coworkers (2) has shown a clearly defined association between GERD symptoms and esophageal cancer. The more frequent, more severe, and longer lasting the reflux symptoms are, the greater the risk. Among patients with long-standing and severe symptoms of reflux, the odds ratio for adenocarcinoma was 43.5. Appropriate endoscopic screening of patients at risk is strongly encouraged.

REFERENCES

1. **Silverstein MD, Patterson T, Talley NJ.** Initial endoscopy with empiric therapy with or without testing for *Helicobacter pylori* for dyspepsia: decision analysis. *Gastroenterology.* 1996; 110:72–83.

2. **Lagergren J, Bergström R, Lindgren A, Nyrén O.** Symptomatic gastroesophageal reflux as a risk factor for esophageal adenocarcinoma. *N Engl J Med.* 1999;340: 825–31.

Index

Reflux, gastroesophageal. *See*
    Gastroesophageal reflux
Regional gastric dysfunction, 33-84
Resistance, bacterial, 71

S

St. John's wort, 162
Saw palmetto, 162
Scintigraphy in motility disorder, 86
Scottish study of *Helicobacter pylori,*
    70-71
Screening for *Helicobacter pylori,* 141,
    144
Self-therapy, 16-17, 115-132
    access to better therapy and, 128-
        130
    background of, 119-121
    herbal preparations for, 126-127
    lifestyle modification in, 126
    over-the-counter drugs in, 121-124,
        121-125
        antacids, 127
        histamine$_2$-receptor antagonist,
            128
        risks of, 128-130
        seeking medical care and, 125
Serologic screening for *Helicobacter
    pylori,* 141, 144
Sexual dysfunction, 111
Short esophagus, surgery on, 55
Side effects of nonprescription drugs,
    128-129
Sphincter, lower esophageal, in hiatal
    hernia, 48
Stomach, dysmotility of, 81-82
Stress, 112
Structural dyspepsia, 5
Sucralfate, 101
Surgery, antireflux, 54-56
Surveys on dyspepsia treatment, 120

T

Temporal epidemiology of
    Helicobacter pylori infection,
    12-13

Testing for *Helicobacter pylori,* 18-19
    cost analysis of, 145-146
Tetracycline, 65
Traditional Chinese herbal medicine
    philosophy of, 161-162
    studies of, 165
    trials of, 167
Transient LES-relaxation gastroe-
    sophageal reflux
    gastric distention in, 49-50
    pathogenesis of, 44
Trial, clinical
    of alternative therapy, 159-172 *See
        also* Alternative therapy
    of anti-*Helicobacter pylori* therapy,
        68-71
    economic analysis and, 137

U

Ulcer, peptic. *see* Peptic ulcer disease
Upper gastrointestinal malignancy, 15-
    16

V

Visceral hypersensitivity in dysmotili-
    ty, 84-85
Vomiting, gastroparesis causing, 8-9
    diseases associated with, 80
    drugs for, 87-90

W

Work-related problems, 110-111
Work-up, diagnostic
    failure to receive reassurance from,
        130
    quality of life and, 113-114